THE POINTING FINGER

Accusation, Addiction and OCD

STEVE HAWKINS

Onwards and Upwards Publishers
Berkeley House, 11 Nightingale Crescent, Leatherhead,
Surrey, KT24 6PD.
www.onwardsandupwards.org

Printed in the UK by 4edge Limited.

ISBN: 978-1-910197-38-7
Typeface: Sabon LT
Graphic design: LM Graphic Design

ABOUT THE AUTHOR

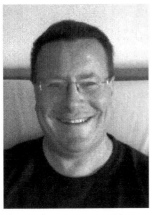

Steve Hawkins teaches English as a Second Language in London and is part of the New Zion Christian Fellowship family in Welwyn Garden City.

Having served the body of Christ for some time, he came to see that he was bound by degrees of legalism, through a visit to Toronto Airport Christian Fellowship. Here he was strongly impacted by the Father's love and now longs to see others enjoy genuine freedom in Jesus Christ.

Previously employed in both the catering and financial services industries, he now teaches students from all over the world in a large college.

The author of 'From Legal to Regal', 'Blood and Glory' and 'The Unbroken Cord: Celebrating Kingdom Sexuality', he ministers today with a growing prophetic edge in leading worship, preaching and teaching.

The author can be contacted at:

steve.hawkins@cheerful.com

Steve longs to see those in the Body of Christ live in the freedom that Jesus has bought on the Cross. If you would like him to speak or minister at an event, please contact him.

"I am allowed to do anything,"
you say. My answer to this is that
not all things are good. Even if it is
true that "I am allowed to do
anything," I will not let anything
control me like a slave.

1 Corinthians 6:12 (ERV)

ACKNOWLEDGEMENTS

Thank you to my parents, friends and church family who have enthusiastically supported my ventures into writing about the power of the Gospel. You remind me that all our ministries truly pertain to the Body of Christ.

I dedicate this book to all those
who have held my hand and
mopped my brow in battles and
skirmishes with accusation. You are
precious people.

Jesus, I acknowledge You as the one
who delivers us from lies into
liberating Truth.

CONTENTS

The Pointing Finger

PREFACE

Let's get straight to the point so that I can tell you what this book is, and what it isn't. You don't want to waste your time or money, after all, do you?

Since the title has attracted you to pick up and open this book; you may be someone who feels that

> Our adversary knows *who* you have become, and are becoming, *whose* you have become, and he fumes that he has lost his authority over you.

they have often been the target of accusation or have perhaps battled some form of addiction; maybe you are an Obsessive Compulsive Disorder (OCD) sufferer, or have concerns that you may be struggling with compulsive behaviour of some kind or are in the regular company of someone who does.

This is a book written to Christians who struggle with feelings of guilt, or with addictive / compulsive behaviours. Generous space is given to OCD as it has been a feature of my own journey – as has major deliverance from it!

Hey, Christian, listen up!

There is a finger pointing at each of us who belong to Jesus. Our adversary knows *who* you have become, and are becoming, *whose* you have become, and he fumes that he has lost his authority over you.

You might want to read that last paragraph again.

In 'The Fight'[1], John White writes about the powers of darkness:

> "Have no delusions about their reality or hostility. But do not fear them. The God inside you terrifies them. They

---

[1] See Bibliography (p.106)

cannot touch you, let alone hurt you. But they can still seduce and they will try."

This book is about identity in the Kingdom of God and looks also at the other kingdom – the kingdom of darkness. My own journey has seen assaults from our adversary's major weapon – *accusation* – and I want to share what I have learned along the way. By God's grace, it's really going to help you!

We also look at the tangles of OCD and how there is a way forward towards freedom. I still encounter a few skirmishes from time to time, BUT the battle has been won. I credit Jesus Christ as my provider and means of newfound freedom.

He's so like that. He does a good job. He reveals (brings reality into the light) in order to heal.

It isn't a biological, systematic analysis in terms of OCD (other authors could probably help you there) although I will share insights I have learned along the way. If you are an OCD slave (sorry – hope that little truth bomb didn't hurt too much), you don't want *information* so much as *revelation*. You need to understand that OCD is based in accusation and is an addiction. Freedom is available.

I share many of my own struggles and trust this information to you transparently with the prayer that it may contribute to your own freedom in Christ and/or to those you care about. Hopefully, my vulnerability will add strength and a helping hand to you.

Accusation and OCD manifest themselves in a variety of expressions, and we will especially concentrate on the issues of *guilt* and *fear*. I will particularly take time to consider the *pointing finger*, a term to describe the infernal one who attempts to load us with condemnation and accusation; this is primarily the area of OCD where I have been captive.

I also want to take a look at the *nature* of addiction; again, I am not a medical practitioner, but there is much I have walked through in this arena, and the ultimate doctor – God – has done a good job in me and would love equally to bring you into freedom.

You will be encouraged and reminded of who you are in Jesus Christ; if you don't know Him, you may be introduced! There is no-one I could more highly recommend you getting to know.

God wants us to be 'whole' people. The provision has been made at the Cross for our restoration, and the job was finished and finished well. God would have us share in the spoils of the war He won. The lid is coming off our lives; we can no longer expect to move on in God as we might wish with hidden bondage remaining untouched.

Freedom

Bondage can only exist through lies, or through the damage of lies.

> GALATIANS 5:1
>
> "It was for freedom that Christ set us free; therefore keep standing firm and do not be subject again to a yoke of slavery."

God's Word translation (GOD'S WORD) puts it like this:

> "Christ has freed us so that we may enjoy the benefits of freedom. Therefore, be firm in this freedom, and don't become slaves again."

It's a wonderful promise to take hold of, that freedom is available in Jesus. The words "do not be subject" suggest a part that we have to play, too. We are going to align ourselves with Jesus and His finished work, and *expect* to live in His abundance, not slavery.

Let's not settle for less.

> "On the Cross Satan was defeated, and although that is by no means the entire significance of the Cross, it does mean that today we can rely with total assurance on that victory. Until the time of final judgement there will inevitably be encounters with the strong man for all of us in our Christian

11

lives, but we should never forget nor be diverted from the fact that *the victory has already been attained.*"[2]

---

[2] Lynda Rose, emphasis added; see Bibliography (p.106)

FOREWORD BY JOHN CAIRNS

In his latest book, Steve seeks to address a major and critical issue faced by many people. The Bible clearly teaches that when we are born again we are adopted into the Family of God, becoming sons and heirs to all the promises of God, through all that Jesus Christ has achieved for us.

We join a family where God, *the* loving Father, desires to positively impact every area of our lives. Yet so many continue to live without a real and genuine awareness of their newfound acceptance and belonging. Christians are filled with the Holy Spirit, who wants to help and empower them to live the life promised in the Word of God.

In his book Steve doesn't give trite and simplistic answers to this issue but genuinely delves into the topic with candour and honesty, continually pointing the way to freedom, acceptance and liberty through Jesus Christ.

John Cairns
President, John Cairns Ministries
International Team leader for Leaders Network International

The Pointing Finger

1

TRUTH: WHO WE ARE IN CHRIST

I could recommend many books to you which wonderfully cover topics such as 'who you have become in Christ Jesus' and our 'new identity' in Him. Colin Urquhart's 'In Christ Jesus' (1997: Kingdom Faith Ministries) is excellent, for example. 'Destined to Reign' (2010: Harrison House) by Joseph Prince brought chain breaking revelation to me at just the time when it was needed.

Although I am not going to consider this in as much detail as those books mentioned above, our new identity is nevertheless an apt place to begin since much of what follows is a look at what is basically *a spiritual attack* on that identity, manifesting itself in our lives as disorder and disordered behaviour.

Your identity in Jesus is certain. Please understand that. In fact, nothing could be any more certain than that. But our beliefs about

> **Your identity in Jesus is certain.**

that identity may be less so. And that can open doors to turbulence.

You don't open the doors of an aircraft flying at 35,000 feet. Since we are seated much higher than that, in heavenly places, we should be especially determined to keep the doors firmly locked! (OK, it's a suspect analogy, but I quite like it!)

Let's just recall and affirm this now: Satan lost his hold on you and me over two thousand years ago. He is insanely jealous of us, and recognising this can shed light on the ferocity of some of the struggles

> Satan lost his hold on you and me over two thousand years ago.

we encounter. Having lost you, he can now only attempt to thwart your progress and spoil your enjoyment of whom you have become in Christ.

Fury

Have you ever been *livid?* I like that word – livid. It's very onomatopoeic, don't you think? It sounds exactly like its meaning. Livid! Jumping mad! So angry you can barely get a word out. You could burst a blood vessel with rage.

That is how angry the enemy is about losing his authority over your life. *He* rebelled against God and was thrown out of paradise. *You* and *I* were born rebels; and while still rebels in nature and behaviour, He drew us to Himself. Praise God!

ROMANS 5:8

"But God demonstrates His own love toward us, in that while we were yet sinners, Christ died for us."

The Message says:

ROMANS 5:8 (THE MESSAGE, EMPHASIS ADDED)

"He didn't, and doesn't, wait for us to get ready. He presented himself for this sacrificial death when we were far *too weak and rebellious* to do anything to get ourselves ready."

Can you imagine living uninterrupted in the glorious presence of the All Glorious One and then leaving that environment? Not only that, but knowing too that you have been banished from it *for ever*, as Satan has been? It is his calamity of calamities, and irreversible, and He is furious.

When we are under spiritual attack there can be a tendency to become passive; to defend and bunker in. In these opening pages we are going to do the opposite; we are going to *intentionally* acknowledge who we are in Jesus Christ and begin to shake off some of the fear and oppression which may have clung to us for a while.

Kingdom Realities

Once upon a time, you and I belonged to a ruler. We were citizens of his domain – for now we will call it a kingdom. We were born into it automatically. Although fashioned in the image of a different king, we were nevertheless born with flaws symptomatic of the first kingdom.

This first kingdom is called Darkness.

It is dark because it lacks light. It lacks the *light of revelation* which brings true understanding. It is dark because it is self-serving and a realm where self and independence are exalted. In this realm there is no revelation of how we were fashioned or to what temporal and eternal purpose. It is impossible to live according to that purpose as a citizen of this first realm, the realm of Darkness. One cannot *live* in the *light* where there is only darkness.

In fact, if true *living* can only take place within the *light*, then you and I cannot really live at all in the realm of Darkness. You can only… exist.

The Bible shows us that we are spirit, soul and body. The latter may be alive, but what about the rest of us? The earthly tent may be erected, but is anyone *living* and breathing at home?

The ruler of the kingdom of darkness does not want to lose his citizens, but he does not have the power to stop someone leaving if they choose to do so. When they leave and become citizens of the other kingdom – there are only two kingdoms, right? – he can only seek to resist, to unsettle them and try to convince them that the old rules, those of Darkness, still apply and that they have not really transferred at all. If that fails, he tries to convince them that they are unworthy to live in the Kingdom of Light and don't truly belong there. He magnifies our shortcomings and failures, and hopes to wear us down and have us wallow in doubt, self-pity and self-recrimination.

Deception

In other words, all he can do is to try to *deceive* us. You deceive people by lying to them and by withholding truth from them.

When someone leaves Darkness and becomes a citizen of the Kingdom of Light, or simply "the Kingdom", a lot changes.

They actually become a new person. Their first nature is superseded by a new one. Although they retain the ability to experience some of the old nature, nevertheless they have received a new nature and they are to live in it. In Jesus, we are *designed* to live from the new nature:

> 2 CORINTHIANS 5:17
>
> "Therefore if anyone is in Christ, he is a new creature; the old things passed away; behold, new things have come."

Part of The Message translation of that verse is as follows:

> "Now we look inside, and what we see is that anyone united with the Messiah gets a fresh start, is created new…"

The New Living Translation (NLT) says that "anyone who belongs to Christ has become a new person…"

Jesus is King of the Kingdom of Light.

The Bible says that the first, old nature was actually killed. It masquerades, at times, as still being alive, but it died when Christ died.

> GALATIANS 2:20 (EMPHASIS ADDED)
>
> I have been *crucified* with Christ and I no longer live, but Christ lives in me. The life I now live in the body, I live by faith in the Son of God, who loved me and gave himself for me.

Living in Light

The new nature lives within the realm of *light*. I will now refer to this light as 'Light' in recognition of Jesus Christ who is the Light. In Light we learn the truth about whom we have become and of what has been left behind. We learn about this new identity as people belonging to a new Kingdom – one ruled by a supreme, magnificent, perfect king, the King of Love. This King is all-powerful and the very nature of love. You could not wish to belong to a more awesome King. He has a tailored purpose for each of our lives.

The King wants us to know His love by getting to know Him and wants us to participate in the redemption of individuals still bound within Darkness. Just as was the case with many of us, they do not understand why there is so much dysfunction in their lives because they have no light, no revelation. Many of them are unable to separate the disorder itself from their own personal identity, indeed, in many respects the two may have become inseparable. Our King wants us to share in the task of bringing them out of this darkness into His Light, where *revelation* flows.

Evangelism may or may not involve talking, explaining and the use of various media and materials, but I believe it is primarily about *modelling* the new Life of Jesus. The power inherent in this is in our allowing God's Presence to express Himself through us. This is far more powerful than us just trying to 'say the right thing' or behave as we think Jesus might act.

I have nothing against the 'What Would Jesus Do?' (WWJD) ethos but would prefer a LWJD ethos, 'Look What Jesus Does!'

Loser

The usurping ruler, whose name is Satan, is not at all happy to lose subjects to the Kingdom. He and his workers seek to oppose the redemptive work, but the King of Light has played His master stroke.

Over two thousand years ago, He wrestled back (following Adam and Eve's capitulation) the authority over people's lives from Satan. Anyone who chooses to transfer to the Kingdom of Light can do so.

Satan has workers (as does the King of Light), Satan's servants seek to misinform, lie and keep people *out of revelation*. These spirit beings (or demons, as they are called) are outnumbered two to one by the King's workers – angels. Angels minister to humans on behalf of the Kingdom of Light and support the church in establishing Kingdom authority on earth. Sometimes angels act in response to a Kingdom agenda unknown to us. At other times, they respond to our prayers and those of others on our behalf.

Demons, also known as unclean spirits, operate in the realm of darkness. They are real spiritual beings with an agenda. In Jesus, however, we need not fear them, rather, we have authority over them.

Unseen Combat

There is a spiritual battle going on for people's lives and destinies. The battle for the Christian's life has been won already. But the enemy will try to impair our effectiveness as an ambassador of the Kingdom of Light. He may try to put sickness or discouragement on you, tempt you to sin or distract you with busyness. He might even try to get you to be excessively busy in the church in the hope that you lose touch with your first love, the King of Light, Jesus. This is not an uncommon line of attack.

Another way that he may try to tackle you is through *accusation*. This may come in the form of verbal attacks from people or it could come through thoughts in your mind. Often, they will arrive on your doorstep as a bolt out of the blue.

Their design and purpose is to harass you and cause you to lose confidence in who you really are in Jesus; to question your identity, to threaten you so that you retreat from pursuing the fullness of what God has for you.

In Jesus, you will always be a son; always loved; always cherished; always accepted; always supported and always provided for. God will always be faithful to you, be present in and with you, and He will always look for opportunities to bless you. He is like that. He is unreservedly for you. He is your greatest fan.

> "Fan: an enthusiastic devotee, follower, or admirer of a sport, pastime, celebrity, etc."[3]

The Living God is a devoted follower of *you* – you are a celebrity in His eyes. But Satan would have you doubt Him and who you are in Him. This jealous accuser has lost you to another, infinitely more powerful than he, and you are now a significant threat to him. As Christ outworks His Kingdom Life in you, you become a greater threat as this power lives and expresses itself through you.

Jesus said that John the Baptist was the least in the Kingdom of Heaven. Consider for a moment how He must regard *you!*

The enemy may try to bind you with addictions or capture your attention with other 'loves'; things which may hold no danger in themselves but which can cause damage when unwisely handled.

Satan, the Accuser of the Brethren, is a defeated opponent, but he has not yet been silenced or bound for ever.

Baggage

So how is it that we are vulnerable to attack?

There are many reasons and, of course, we are all unique; we come to Jesus with an absolutely unique history, with unique, unwanted baggage and as flawed souls. Christ comes to inhabit us by the Holy Spirit, and we then have to learn to live from our redeemed spirit, that new creation, rather than the 'programme' that has been running us previously.

---

[3] http://dictionary.reference.com/browse/fan

Family trees are all different and there have been unique spiritual inputs (from both kingdoms); many have been damaged by the presence or absence of key influential individuals.

We have made our mistakes, perhaps pushed a proverbial domino down that set off a chain of related incidents and consequences. Events have conspired, at times, to convince us that we were hopeless, useless, destined to fail. Some of us have been slow to learn from our mistakes, repeating them and inflicting grief upon ourselves and others.

It is worth remembering that...

ROMANS 5:8

"God demonstrates His own love toward us, in that while we were yet sinners, Christ died for us."

Part of The Message translation reads:

ROMANS 5:8 (THE MESSAGE)

"He didn't, and doesn't, wait for us to get ready. He presented himself for this sacrificial death when we were far too weak and rebellious to do anything to get ourselves ready. And even if we hadn't been so weak, we wouldn't have known what to do anyway."

We arrived at the doors of the Kingdom as flawed, grubby people. And despite the fact that we have been made new creations in Jesus Christ, there is much to un-learn for some of us; there are principles that we have lived by which are not Kingdom of Light principles; we need to be transformed by the renewing of our minds and begin to see that Kingdom principles work in the Kingdom and – indeed – they are much more effective at bringing about transformation into wholeness than those old ones that have been part of our thinking, psyche and experience for a long time.

God is the Author and Finisher of our faith and is committed to the transforming work He is doing in each of our lives; to transform us into the likeness of Jesus and, in so doing, into who you and I were really designed to be.

We have received a new identity, one that is going to be the basis for our flourishing and progress in the Kingdom of Light.

But at times we have to contend for it because the Accuser will contest it.

Truth Food

Some truth for you to 'ponder' ("Selah"):

EPHESIANS 2:4-7 (EMPHASIS ADDED)

"But God, being rich in mercy, because of His great love with which He loved us, even when we were dead in our transgressions, made us alive together with Christ [by grace you have been saved], and raised us up with Him, and seated us with Him in the heavenly *places* in Christ Jesus, so that in the ages to come He might show the surpassing riches of His grace in kindness toward us in Christ Jesus. For by grace you have been saved through faith; and that not of yourselves, *it is* the gift of God; not as a result of works, so that no one may boast."

1 JOHN 1:9

"If we confess our sins, He is faithful and righteous to forgive us our sins and to cleanse us from all unrighteousness."

ROMANS 5:1

"Therefore, having been justified by faith, we have peace with God through our Lord Jesus Christ..."

1 PETER 1:17-21 (EMPHASIS ADDED)

"If you address as Father the One who impartially judges according to each one's work, conduct yourselves in fear during the time of your stay *on earth;* knowing that you were not redeemed with perishable things like silver or gold from your futile way of life inherited from your forefathers, but with precious blood, as of a lamb unblemished and spotless, the blood of Christ. For He was foreknown before the foundation of the world, but has appeared in these last times for the sake of you who through Him are believers in God, who raised Him from the dead and gave Him glory, so that your faith and hope are in God."

2 CORINTHIANS 5:14

"For the love of Christ controls us, having concluded this, that one died for all, therefore all died..."

GALATIANS 2:20 (EMPHASIS ADDED)

"I have been crucified with Christ; and it is no longer I who live, but Christ lives in me; and the *life* which I now live in the flesh I live by faith in the Son of God, who loved me and gave Himself up for me."

COLOSSIANS 3:3

"For you have died and your life is hidden with Christ in God."

ROMANS 6:27

"...for he who has died is freed from sin."

1 CORINTHIANS 1:30

"But by His doing you are in Christ Jesus, who became to us wisdom from God, and righteousness and sanctification, and redemption..."

1 CORINTHIANS 6:11

"Such were some of you; but you were washed, but you were sanctified, but you were justified in the name of the Lord Jesus Christ and in the Spirit of our God."

ROMANS 12:4-5

"For just as we have many members in one body and all the members do not have the same function, so we, who are many, are one body in Christ, and individually members one of another."

Where Are We?

There are some glorious truths here about our identity, and I pray that the Holy Spirit will speak them to you in a far more lasting, impacting way than I am able to! It is important for us to focus on Jesus and who we are in Him – later we will look at some of the characteristics, weaponry and lines of attack of the Accuser, but our best form of attack and defence is to assert and affirm our new identities and live as sons who, as we have just read in Ephesians 2, have been placed / positioned / seated with Christ in the heavenly places, far *above* all rule and authority. We are not living to reach that place; we live *from* there because that is where we already are in Jesus!

We are forgiven, justified (JUST as IF I'D never sinned), washed in a Blood like no other; we were crucified (killed) with Him on the Cross so that now we live as a new creation, a new person, in-filled with the Spirit of God. This is who we are!

I love the last verse I have given you from Romans 12; comparing ourselves with others is fairly pointless seeing that God says that we are all individually gifted in different functions in this amazing Body of Christ. You cannot compare a 'one-off' as there is nothing or no-one to compare them with!

The Holy Spirit wants to bring Kingdom revelation to our lives. He wants to help us get to know the Father, Jesus and *Him, the Holy Spirit*. The Holy Spirit is a person whom we can partner with and build relationship with. We are not to simply 'use' Him as a power source; He deserves our love, respect and the investment of our time in getting to genuinely know Him.

2

LOVE DEFICITS

Having arrived in the new Kingdom as a new creation, yet one with many habits and memories of the previous realm, its ways and its management, God would have us really 'come home'.

JOHN 14:6

"Jesus said to him, 'I am the way, and the truth, and the life; no one comes to the Father but through Me.'"

You see, I don't think a lot of new Christians really come home for a while. Some may not have really arrived 'home' at all, experientially. The verse above is so well known, isn't it? I think we are quite good with the first part – "Jesus is the way" – but less so with the latter part.

The way to where?

It isn't just about 'getting saved', as we tend to think of it. The verse says that there is a destination, that Jesus is the way *to the Father*.

This is the Father that has given His only Son so that you and I may be redeemed – redeemed *into* an entirely new relationship. This is the Father who gave up His precious one because He considered you and me to be worth acquiring as sons. This is the Father who set the deal up even while we were still sinners and a long way off the notion of coming home.

We were not only transferred out of a realm but very intentionally moved into another.

I believe that there are many Christians in the Body of Christ with an *orphan mentality* because they have not yet had a revelation of the love and acceptance of the Father. I imagine that some of them simply "don't want to go there" because of unpleasant experiences with their natural father; or they are apathetic because 'father' just doesn't really attract them as a concept worthy of exploration. This is understandable if their earthly dad has/had been largely absent or passive; or, put another way, if the *reality of authentic relationship* lacked worth to them.

You can be saved and living in Christ, filled with the Holy Spirit and operating in ministry – and still not really know the Father. But we can only effectively minister from what we have from God, from whom we have genuinely become. I can give you words about such-and-such a subject, but the anointing is strong when it is about something that I have walked through and been transformed in.

This kind of 'functional faith walk' may have been a common characteristic through a family for years – even through generations. It is as if we have been given the keys to the house, as sons and daughters, and yet some of us have been content to remain in the hallway, never really enjoying the comforts of the house, of the family, and of the Father of the house. Maybe we never knew that the building had more rooms.

Sometimes we have to contend for what is ours in Jesus Christ. We have to sit up or stand up, acknowledge where we have not tasted something of the Kingdom's fullness and where we have been robbed and say, "No! I am not having or settling for this in my life!"

We may need to say, "Yes – this peace that He gives is mine! Peace and rest are mine in Christ! However I may have lived previously, and however my dad and grandfather may have been, I am standing on the Word of God which says that I am a new creation, that old things have gone and that these disorders have no place in me!"

We don't have to rant and rave, but we need to be proactive. Our authority is not in shouting and screaming, but in affirming and owning what Jesus has done and whom Jesus has made us, in Him.

Some people like to be loud, but loud is not necessarily effective! Others are very measured but the anointing on and through them breaks yokes that bind people and situations. This is a spiritual deal – it's all about *Who* you know, if you get what I mean!

Self-medication

We can do a lot, ourselves, to restore some of the deficits that we may have been living in. We may need to begin to undo some of the *self-medicating* behaviours which we have engaged in. Some people eat a lot, or bury themselves into TV, or become subservient to sexual or other forms of stimulation as a means of masking or numbing a deep, inner pain. The problem is that the desire for that 'pleasure hit' can very quickly master us if we are not alert to its devices. Full blown addiction can result so it's always good to ask the Holy Spirit to shine His light on our 'hidden' heart.

God would have us bring these things into the light, maybe with the help of a trusted, balanced, reliable believer.

If we do not address deficits in our lives, then these areas can become landing strips for the enemy. He has nothing good to give us, however attractive it might seem to be. Anything that comes our way from his storehouse will surely have a sting in its tail, sooner or later. He is like the child catcher in 'Chitty Chitty Bang Bang', promising treats in order to lure the naïve into imprisonment.

Jesus wants us to experience His abundance and His generosity. That is the surest way to enable us to drop some of our substitute desires and behaviours.

I appreciate that some of the bondage that plagues us may be deep-seated. Some of us may be receiving – and need to continue to receive – professional help with regard to physical, mental or emotional issues.

You know... that's all right! God, your and my amazing Father, is not fazed by the road we have taken; He knows how and why we are where we are. And wherever that place may be, be it on glorious heights or in miserable depths, He is right on our case, looking to bless us, heal and restore us. He is not disappointed in you or me.

I said, *He is not disappointed in you.* As Graham Cooke sometimes says, God cannot be in any way disillusioned with you because He had no illusions about you in the first place.

Keep Psalm 139 in mind. He knows you intimately, cell by cell. He is thrilled that you are His. He is proud to be your heavenly Dad.

Graham Cooke writes:

> "The love of God is never less than 100%. He just doesn't know how to be otherwise. He is unchanging and consistent. He takes joy in the fact that He is the Lord and that He never changes. He is the same yesterday, today and forever; we can be confident of who He is for us."[4]

However, someone else sees your blessing and holds a grudge.

---

[4] Graham Cooke; see Bibliography (p.106)

3

THE ACCUSER

REVELATION 12:10 (EMPHASIS ADDED)

"Then I heard a loud voice in heaven, saying, 'Now the salvation, and the power, and the kingdom of our God and the authority of His Christ have come, *for the accuser of our brethren has been thrown down, he who accuses them before our God day and night.*'"

Now there's an insight! Satan, having lost his dominion over you as a born again believer, constantly tries to swipe back at you with accusation. Look how relentless he is! The Amplified Bible gives part of the verse above thus:

REVELATION 12:10 (AMP, EMPHASIS ADDED)

"...for the accuser of our brethren, *he who keeps bringing before our God charges against them day and night,* has been cast out!"

The Holy Spirit wants to, equally consistently, affirm you as the new creature, the new person you have become in Jesus. He wants to affirm the finished work of the Cross which has moved you out of Darkness, into the Kingdom of Light. He wants to remind us that our acceptance and innocence are not due to our performance but due to what Jesus did on the Cross. He wants us to come into a place of rest – Holy Spirit rest – where we relax into our identity and live from it, rather than strive to attain it.

We cannot attain something we have already been given! If we have been given it, we have it. Would you continue to ask me for a piece of chocolate cake if I had already given it to you on a plate? I guess you would only ask if you didn't know the cake was already in your possession.

The Accuser knows who you are, and the only card he has left to play is to lie to you. He wants to tie us up in guilt and compulsive, addictive behaviours which can delay us from entering into all that God has purposed for us to enjoy. God has appointed us to enjoy the quality of our lives. Freedom has been purchased for us, and the Accuser knows this. Holy Spirit freedom means that we are not mastered by blessing but enjoy it in His right order.

The Accuser wants to attack your confidence and your self-esteem. He tries to engage you in a tiring, extensive programme of self-analysis. The Holy Spirit does not do such a thing. He loves to engage us in attention to Jesus, to His finished work and to whom we have now become in the Kingdom of Heaven.

When we look at what the Bible says about our enemy, we learn that, despite how it may feel at times, there really is no contest when we consider our Saviour.

B-i-g Mistake

Lucifer made a calamitous misjudgement.

He, equally, makes a similar error of judgement when he seeks to harass and persecute you and me. God takes everything he does and mixes it perfectly into the pot of our redemption, using it and transforming it for our Kingdom benefit.

Lucifer lived in the glory. He was a glorious being, too. God had created him. How could he not be glorious? But somehow, within that sin-free realm, pride was found within Lucifer's will. He abused that will, chose to exalt himself and chose to challenge the All Glorious God who had created him. And he paid dearly and very finally for it.

Chess

I remember hearing a speaker way back when I was at Birmingham University. He described the dispute between Lucifer and God as a chess match.

Do you play, or have you played, chess? I quite enjoy the occasional game although I tire easily – especially against a better player! It's always the same problem – apart from the fact that I'm probably just not very good. My opponent is *ahead of me*. He can see several moves ahead and strategise accordingly. I try to play a sweeping, conclusive move (usually much too early on in the proceedings) while my superior opponent responds with an almost unnoticed, subtle one which turns out to be the *key move*.

God has never been outwitted, and He dealt with Lucifer effectively, casting him out. And at just the right time, Jesus came, died and rose again to win back the authority that Adam had lost. We do well to remind ourselves, also, that God is as much in control concerning the end game as He was in the beginning. It may seem like the enemy has had too much access to us, to our loved ones and probably beyond those family relationships too. Nevertheless, the Father, Son and Holy Spirit are the Chess Master. The key moves have been made, and they have, too, in our lives. We have been placed, through the Blood of Jesus, on to the Rock that is Christ.

ISAIAH 28:16

"Therefore thus says the Lord God, 'Behold, I am laying in Zion a stone, a tested stone, a costly cornerstone for the foundation, firmly placed. He who believes in it will not be disturbed.'"

The word "disturbed" in this verse means "in a hurry" or "moved by panic". This foundation is not going to budge in our lives; we need to stay in His rest and walk it out.

Having been made alive in Jesus, we are now more open to, and aware of, the spiritual realm than we were when we were citizens of Darkness.

Remember, we have much more than a hotline to heaven. We live *from* heaven!

So, our adversary, unable to touch our position, can only attempt to harass us by various means.

Seeing our hunger and love for Jesus, he tries to muddy the waters. Whether we like it or not, we are now actively opposed to him and a major threat to his power base. We want to please our wonderful Saviour; in fact, He is already delighted in us as His own! Isn't it because we are His that we want to pursue Him?

So Satan tries to meddle with our blossoming relationship with Jesus. I am sure, at some time or another, we have all encountered, and had to deal with, doubts that may assail us concerning our lives and how they are working out. The adversary will try to attack our Father's character and then get us to agree with him! We may face challenges in the family, in the workplace or in our finances.

Tactics

The Accuser is anti-Christ and anti-Cross. He works diametrically opposed to the Kingdom of Heaven.

Thus, he will have you believe that the Cross is *not* a finished work; that you are still not good enough; that you have to do more to gain God's acceptance; that you are not spiritual enough.

He will try to distract you with 'other' things. He may try to load you with a sense of responsibility (false responsibility) for someone or something which God would not have you give time and energy to. We will discuss this in further detail later.

A major line of assault is through firing condemnation at us. We need to look at this.

4

CONDEMNATION – THE FAKE CONVICTION

"What is your vision of God? How you see Him is how you see yourself ... If you fail to see Jesus as your Prince of Peace, that may be why you cannot find any rest. Seeing Him as your personal Prince of Peace means you're not allowed to worry anymore; peace and worry cannot co-exist. The way we live is profoundly shaped by our vision of God."[5]

Desiring to grow in an intimate relationship with Jesus, we are going to encounter some spiritual dynamics; it's interesting how we learn and grow because no two believers really walk the same road. It may seem as though there are many similarities, but actually there are dynamics that I encountered very early in my Christian life that, I know, others have not seen yet. And vice versa, absolutely!

In the heavenly realms you and I are known. We are sealed into Jesus; we bear the mark of his ownership. I don't know exactly what that looks like but, having transferred kingdoms, this has not gone unnoticed in the heavenlies!

We are invited to expect to live in Jesus' abundance. This is our new birthright. Such an overflowing life achieves much fruit in the Kingdom so the enemy tries to weigh us down with guilt and condemnation in an effort to have us keep a distance from our Father's presence.

---

[5] Graham Cooke

But maybe I have done something wrong and *should* feel guilty. Maybe God is trying to teach me a lesson – because I certainly deserve it!

Hang on, hang on! This is the kind of bewitching nonsense which Paul writes to the Galatian church about, warning them about this line of attack.

GALATIANS 3:1-3

"You foolish Galatians, who has bewitched you, before whose eyes Jesus Christ was publicly portrayed as crucified? This is the only thing I want to find out from you: did you receive the Spirit by the works of the Law, or by hearing with faith? Are you so foolish? Having begun by the Spirit, are you now being perfected by the flesh?"

It is easy, tempting, to fall back into those bad habits. Is our standing in Jesus secure because of our own efforts? Has that ever been the case? Graham Cooke posted the following onto the social networking site Facebook in August 2013:

"The faithfulness of God is established in and through the person of Christ. Heaven is open to us. Performance is dead. Placement is everything. As we live up to our position in Christ, we will receive every blessing available to Him."

Performance is dead; placement is everything. This can be life-changing for us! It is a magnificent revelation and an effective weapon against enemy accusation.

> **Performance is dead; placement is everything.**

Each time the enemy accuses us that we are unworthy to enjoy God's presence because of something that we have actually, or supposedly, done, we need to look past the pointing finger to the Cross.

The Holy Spirit's role in our lives is to express Jesus to us and then through us. You know these verses, I am sure, from John 16:

JOHN 16:7-11

"But I tell you the truth, it is to your advantage that I go away; for if I do not go away, the Helper will not come to you; but if I go, I will send Him to you. And He, when He comes, will convict the world concerning sin and righteousness and judgement; concerning sin, because they do not believe in Me; and concerning righteousness, because I go to the Father and you no longer see Me; and concerning judgement, because the ruler of this world has been judged."

I was always concerned that my guilty feelings came from the Holy Spirit; that He was convicting me of my sinfulness, saying, "Steve, you missed the mark again. Look what you did! You need to repent and make it right or you will be separated from God."

We are now sons.

The Scripture says something very different. The Holy Spirit convicts us of sin and we come to Jesus, confessing our need of Him and we receive Him as our Lord and Saviour. Then, the Holy Spirit convicts us of our *righteousness in Jesus*. He already convicted us of our sin; we responded to Him and embraced the work of the Cross in our lives. We are now sons, adopted into God's family and in right standing with Him. If we do fall into sin, we respond by acknowledging our righteousness in Jesus. We get up, brush ourselves down, and get on with living with Jesus. When He disciplines us, as He sometimes does, it is not a spiteful response but a liberating affirmation! Satan would have us constantly examining ourselves to see if we measure up and endlessly confessing our shortcomings. Well, God already measured us and has found that we measure up in the image of His Son, Jesus Christ. He measured us and we fit into Jesus just fine!

If that sounds too good to be true – you know, *surely* His grace cannot be that good – then this Scripture helps:

ROMANS 2:4 (EMPHASIS ADDED)

Or do you think lightly of the riches *of His kindness* and tolerance and patience, not knowing that the *kindness of God* leads you to repentance?

I have found this to be true in my life, that it is knowing His kindness that transforms me and changes my desires. Rules and self-imposed laws have a very limited shelf life, in my experience. In fact, they feed my flesh because I feel that I am doing something to improve myself. The reality is that my resolutions to 'do better' only seem to bridle my sin nature and its behaviours for a short time. It is only by walking in the Spirit that we overcome and 'reckon' the flesh nature to be dead.

GALATIANS 5:16

"But I say, walk by the Spirit, and you will not carry out the desire of the flesh."

The Message says:

GALATIANS 5:16-18

"My counsel is this: Live freely, animated and motivated by God's Spirit. Then you won't feed the compulsions of selfishness. For there is a root of sinful self-interest in us that is at odds with a free spirit..."

"Oh Steve, you just want to have it easy; you don't deserve such kindness." There's that Accuser again. True, I don't deserve it; but yes, I absolutely welcome it and receive it and stand upon it.

So, this condemnation that comes our way is illegal! Christ has fulfilled the law, and you and I are *not guilty.*

Now – we want Holy Spirit to speak to us, to lead us and we certainly don't want to avoid His discipline, which we mentioned earlier, because being corrected and taught is part of being a son. However, on occasions the enemy likes to masquerade as the Holy Spirit. How can we identify who is speaking?

I remember clearly wanting a formula for this one.

How can you tell the difference between the Holy Spirit's conviction and the enemy's condemnation? If I'm honest I never really found anyone else's answer quite did it for me. I would read or hear something like: "Condemnation brings a general sense of guilt and unworthiness, whilst the Holy Spirit is always very specific about what He wants to speak to us about."

But what if you frequently feel guilty about very specific things? Basically I believed for years that the taunts aimed at me *had to be* the Holy Spirit because they didn't appear to be my own natural thoughts and *were so specific.*

My Crucial Discovery

So here's how it works for me.

I now know that, having come to Jesus, the Holy Spirit's job of convicting me of sin has been accomplished. In Christ, He now convicts me of my righteousness. Relating to me as His son, His firm but kind discipline helps me to grow; it's actually fun! I am affirmed and loved in His dealings. If and when I do something inappropriate (or conversely, fail to speak, think or act appropriately), the Holy Spirit shows me so. It's empowering, positive and I feel gratitude for His involvement.

"Steve! This is who you really are! You are a man after My heart; you are peaceable and respectful; you are gentle and move in purity…"

On the other hand, the enemy deals in fear and accusation. When he is at work, when he gets involved to make a judgement upon me, to point his finger at me, it causes me to be disturbed, upset, bringing a sense of dread and self-recrimination.

"Look what you did! How appalling! You'll never make it in God's Kingdom. You might as well pack it in! A *real* Christian wouldn't have done/said that. You just bring disgrace to God! You're a hypocrite and a liar. If people really knew what you were like…"

Jesus said:

MATTHEW 7:15-20

"Beware of the false prophets, who come to you in sheep's clothing, but inwardly are ravenous wolves. You will know them by their fruits. Grapes are not gathered from thorn bushes nor figs from thistles, are they? So every good tree bears good fruit, but the bad tree bears bad fruit. A good tree cannot produce bad fruit, nor can a bad tree produce good fruit. Every tree that does not bear good fruit is cut down and thrown into the fire. So then, you will know them by their fruits."

The Message describes the "false prophets" as diseased trees with their bad apples.

A prophet 'proclaims'. That is what the enemy does. He proclaims and it's all lies! As we look at the fruit – compare the fruit as I have described it above – the source of the mouth speaking becomes very evident.

A friend of mine, Peter, really helped me here. He really encouraged me to look at the fruit! I am so grateful to him because I saw that I had been listening to lies for – well – years and years.

I had even made some fairly major decisions based on the premise that "God must be telling me to…" when, in fact, it had never been Him at all. You can maybe appreciate, some of these circumstances had produced no little pain. I had made some sacrifices apparently demanded of me by God – but it hadn't been Him.

You see, I had wanted to please Him. But pleasing someone that you love is a different dynamic to trying to please – or placate – someone that you are afraid of.

I want to please the Lord now in a very different manner. Firstly, I know that He is already pleased – in fact, delighted – with me! He thinks I'm great! I'm His! Also, I am not afraid he will be displeased with me because I know how He feels about me. Rather, I want to bless

God because I love Him. I want to obey His Holy Spirit and fulfil my life in Him because we love each other. And, if I do slip up and fall into sin, I am not afraid of God. I welcome His correction and encouragement and run into Him!

5

OCD: FUNNY OR NO JOKE?

Let's return to the matter of OCD.

I do actually think that we all need to learn to laugh at ourselves a lot more. Things can get pretty heavy if we don't. Especially as we live in such a 'precious' public society these days. You know what I mean; you can't sniff for the fear of offending someone, or, perhaps more accurately, being told that you are going to do so.

This 'over-care' about being sensitive to one another has the appearance of wisdom, but in reality I think it can stifle us and blanket us with mediocrity and suffocation.

Sometimes those preaching the loudest about tolerance appear to me to be some of the most *intolerant* people on the planet.

Actually I don't really believe that the vast majority are likely to be offended. Nine times out of ten, I don't think anyone is offended at all. Of course, I understand that there is legitimate value in encouraging one another to be sensitive to each other's frailties, but we do need to lighten up. The politically correct agenda thrust at us these days can get very tedious, and no less joy-sapping.

Yes, we are all flawed. We get it. We're just flawed *differently*. Our sense of humour is what, at times, eases the burden and the weight of

> We're just flawed differently.

our various quirks. Our weaknesses can be both amusing and endearing.

When we are in relationship with others, we can bring them priceless support in the way that we respond to their particular struggles. We know, don't we, that we have breathed a sigh of relief when someone that we trust shows us that we, personally, are loved and accepted despite a somewhat embarrassing vulnerability (at least, it appears so in our eyes) that we are prone to.

OCD in its various forms can have a massive effect on the sufferer's life. Society may trivialise the 'behaviour' or 'weakness', but as much as we can support the individual with our patience and good humour, the battle is yet there to be won.

As I discovered, I had to win my battle. I had to approach it, look the demon in the eyes and advance against it. Others held my hands but my own feet had to move forward.

At some stage, the OCD-er who simply has to touch everything equally with his or her left and right hand must be brought face to face with the lie that nourishes such behaviour. They may skirt the problem by shaking your hand with both of theirs at the same time, but it is clear that the behaviour only reinforces the fear that empowers it. It is no easy confrontation, as essential as it will be if the OCD-er is going to break free. The sense of dread is palpable, the heavy weight of responsibility absolutely real. The demand to obey the compulsion, at some stage, must be denied, despite the physical and emotional discomfort experienced.

You get the picture; such struggles could raise some amusement.

"Steve, How Could You?"

Sometimes I mislay things. I say 'mislay' because I don't want to use the word 'lose'. At least 'mislay' suggests retrieval of an item, whilst 'lose' has a sad finality about it.

I remember going on a school trip in my very early teens. Guess who, amongst all the pupils on the trip, lost their boarding pass and held everyone up? I bet you can't.

I used to live in Ongar, an old Tudor market town in Essex, and went to school near Loughton, which is also in Essex but borders the outskirts of Greater London. This meant that I had to use the London Underground train service from Ongar (which was at the end of the Central Line back then) to Epping, change there (by running over a bridge) and continue on another two or three stops.

One day, I had to take my clarinet to school for band practice – as well as my other gear, of course. I got on the train at Ongar and reached Epping. As usual, I joined the melee of early morning commuters as we scrambled over the bridge. I sat down in the carriage and realised that I had left my instrument on the first train.

Leaping up I forced my way back over the bridge, swimming against a tide of passengers moving in the opposite direction. Re-entering the carriage I had arrived in, I recovered my abandoned clarinet before 'legging' it back over the bridge, back on to the waiting train.

Two stops later I got off the second train and left my clarinet on it.

You couldn't make it up. Aren't you glad that you haven't done anything as silly as that? It's alright, I'm not looking your way…

I am a lecturer in a Further Education college in London. Each college year I get to work with four or five groups of up to twenty learners. You get to know them a little bit. As an English teacher, I might have ten to fifteen different nationalities in one class. I love that. So, there are national quirks as well as the individual ones. People are funny. They make me laugh and I try to make them laugh. People learn well with humour and relax when they sense they are accepted.

I like discovering my learners' different personalities and seeing them grow; quiet ones blossom and brash ones become softer and more rounded. I like it that I learn how they are going to react in their range of expressions. I suppose I feel a little bit like a dad.

The world of comedy can have a field day with OCD. Some of the behaviour which results from the syndrome is quite funny. Don't worry, you will get to hear some of my own rather head-scratching activity.

OCD is no joke.

But for many OCD sufferers, OCD is no joke, actually. The same goes for those near and dear to them. They have to put up with a lot. There isn't a lot of fun in the world of fear, and this is the realm where OCD operates. It's a realm we need to plunder because Jesus has already done so, and His authority supersedes that of fear. Having been placed with Christ, far above all rule and authority, we need to have an expectation to see walls of fear begin to shake and indeed come down. Jesus came to open the doors to abundance.

OCD is a compulsive disorder; in basic terms, the OCD sufferer assumes an enormous level of responsibility by believing that they must ensure that a situation is *just right*. For some OCD-ers, they have a fear of something adverse happening, so they feel the absolute need to try to prevent this possibility of the fear becoming a real nightmare. To him (or her), this fear is very real and – more accurately – so much so that omitting to carry out the preventative / corrective behaviour is too painful / terrifying to contemplate.

Trying to tell the OCD sufferer that his fears are groundless is like speaking Italian to a Russian. One author entitled his supportive book 'Brainlock'[6]. That's a good description. It's as if the signals which generally tell you and I that a fear / suggestion is groundless (or unrealistic so that we may dismiss it) somehow get blocked or re-routed. A distant possibility of an event – very distant – becomes a 'round the corner' catastrophe, on the brink of actually happening.

The vicious circle is that the OCD-er tends to believe that it is his personal intervention that prevents the disaster, hence he is bound to believe it is also his responsibility next time too. Ultimately, he needs

---

[6] Jeffery Schwartz; see Bibliography (p.106)

to be shown that he does not need to act – there was going to be no disaster in the first place. It was a *mirage of the mind*. Hmm... Many fears – *most* fears – turn out to be that, don't you agree?

Imagine something ridiculous. I tell you that world peace is dependent upon my diet. Steve Hawkins' diet. That's all. As long as I eat a strawberry yoghurt every evening, there will be no nuclear war.

If I sincerely believe that to be the case, imagine my discomfort at the prospect of not eating a yoghurt. Imagine my agony were I to be confined in such a way so that access to strawberry yoghurt were impossible. Your disbelief at my suggestion does not, in itself, touch my inner turmoil and sense of threat.

This is the 'felt' fear that OCD-ers can experience, however ridiculous it may sound to the rest of us. It is kind of quirky but, believe me, hugely painful for the individual concerned.

Let's take a look at some of those OCD flavours.

6

OCD: WHAT'S IT LIKE FOR YOU?

Having got this far, you probably can relate to aspects of the title of this book in some way or another.

If it is the acronym 'OCD' which grabbed your attention, let's go there. Which OCD traits can you relate to?

Here are some examples of OCD behaviour. A little later, I need to qualify some of the examples because the behaviour itself may not always be evidence of OCD.

For example, you may be a very tidy person; you like to have things neat and ordered in your home. There's nothing wrong with that. But if you experience a compulsion to rearrange, to tidy – in other words, if you feel very uncomfortable about *not* doing so – it may be a sign of OCD-related behaviour.

You don't have to tell me which one is the monkey on your back, or on the back of someone you care about, but do you recognise any of these?

- All the tins in your food cupboard *must* face the front.

- You regularly wash your hands or try to avoid touching surfaces for fear of contamination.

- You regularly have to check several times if you locked that door, window or your car.

- Having walked on the left side of the street, you have to walk on the other side too, to balance things up.

- You dare not drop any litter, especially a food item, on the street. Someone could pick it up and by touching it, or consuming it, become ill. This would then be *your* fault.

- Thoughts come into your head that you hate someone – or love someone. You are afraid of the consequences of acting on these thoughts.

- You tell someone something and then have the thought that you perhaps exaggerated or lied. You feel the need to 'undo' the comment by either apologising or by explaining that you exaggerated or lied.

- You feel compelled to do one good deed after another, because the last one was not quite good enough to satisfy a deep sense of guilt you carry.

- You start counting in your head and only allow yourself to stop when you have reached a certain number. If you miss any numbers out, you make yourself start again.

These are just examples, and I trust you appreciate that the uniqueness of an individual's own behaviours could add a thousand and one variations.

A theme which runs through many if not all of these descriptions is *exactness*. And that involves a lot of *checking*.

Do you want to know what it was like for me? All right, read on. Seat belts on, please!

7

MY OWN BATTLE

I do not particularly know why these tendencies have been in my life. It is true that I seemed to become hooked into a rather legalistic view of God and that this may have contributed. This is peculiar to me because having 'got saved' I entered into free, charismatic-style church environments. You wouldn't have thought that legalism would have been a particular issue for me, would you?

Maybe the wires just became twisted for me. In fact, being part of such a free church set up (and I include here too my first experiences at my university's Christian Union in Birmingham) encouraged me to go for God *to the max!* Suddenly, in Jesus the sky was the limit! Well, not even the sky was the limit! God had a plan for my life, and I didn't want to miss it. I wanted all of it!

What if? What if?

But my insecurities were laid bare; what if I missed it? Yes, what if I missed the great 'It'? What if I took wrong paths? What if I was a deaf sheep? What if? What if? The prizes in Jesus were so monumental that the prospect of somehow flunking haunted me. I certainly did have a fear of displeasing Him or of 'missing the mark', of not being committed enough to Him. I was also afraid of making a mess of my 'calling' through being double-minded, for example.

I suppose I used to be quite double-minded but, on reflection, I'm not so sure. That was a joke, by the way!

I did not really have a healthy view of the Lord, despite being part of a charismatic stream which sought the Holy Spirit and His revelation fervently.

I am so grateful to Him for taking me aside for a while when He began to reveal to me more of His true nature. He did that when I took time out to go to Toronto Airport Christian Fellowship in 2003. I am grateful to God for that place and for those giving, caring people.

But – back to the OCD theme… At the time that I became unwell (or should I say, became aware of my difficulties), I had not really appreciated that on many occasions previously, over the years, an underlying current of malfunction – latent OCD, if you like – had been operating. I have come to realise that these behaviours stemmed from the same pot.

I distinctly remember the following incidents / tendencies:

- If I turned round in an anticlockwise circle, I just *had* to do the same in the opposite direction.

- Making myself hold my breath for a self-imposed length of time.

- Feeling guilty about either impure or negative thoughts and feeling the need to confess. (I'm not saying that impurity doesn't matter. The *fear* that haunted me was a tell-tale sign.)

And a little later in life:

- Worrying if my car door touched the paintwork of a neighbouring vehicle and I saw a scratch on it. I would be afraid that I had caused it and feel the need to mention it to the owner of that vehicle.

- Returning to an office to check that I had locked the back door. I did this on multiple occasions; once, I was half way around the North Circular Road (for you Londoner locals!) when I felt compelled to go back to check.

More recently, as the condition came to a head in my life:

- Feeling the need to apologise to someone for something I said, as it may have implied something I didn't mean. Feeling accused / guilty for having (perhaps) lied or exaggerated or – and I can only describe it this way – *not having told it right.*

- Forcing myself to do things (such as confront someone on an issue) that I was afraid of, as this is how I could prove to God that I was not yielding to fear.

Compulsion

The word 'compelled' is worth considering. Christians use this word a lot when describing the work of the Holy Spirit: "I was shopping in a supermarket and saw this mum with two boisterous children. She was clearly upset and having difficulty in controlling them. I just felt *compelled* to go up to her and encourage her, to tell her…"

What I came to learn, however, is that Holy Spirit leading is not… not… NOT… the same as the enemy's *compulsions*. I have learned that they *feel* completely different. One provokes you with a sense of excitement and compassion; the other accuses you with a sense of dread.

We are going to return to this in a little while. Before that, let's consider in detail the consequences for the OCD-er of *not* following through with their compulsions.

What if you *don't* shake someone by the hand, grasping their hand with both of yours?

What if one of your magazines *is* allowed to lay upside down on your coffee table?

What if you *don't* go back to the church hall to check if you locked up, or if you *don't* go home in the middle of the drama session to check if you really did switch off your hair straighteners?

What might happen if you *did* smack your young son when he is naughty, despite the fact that you are convinced that you will cause him internal injuries and/or permanently damage him psychologically?

8

WHAT WILL HAPPEN IF I DON'T?

Nothing.

Now, please read this chapter again, thank you.

9

PARDON? WHAT WILL REALLY HAPPEN IF I DON'T?

Really, nothing.

Now, there are many books which, through the practice of Cognitive Behaviour Therapy (CBT), can guide you / OCD-ers through examples, explanation and specific activation exercises which will, eventually, prove to you that nothing drastic or negative is going to occur because you *dare* to deny the accusing voice in your head.

I understand that it is a challenge to deny it. You are face to face, eyeball to eyeball with the fear that is binding you; but you are also on the brink of deliverance.

> You are ... eyeball to eyeball with the fear...

This is hand to hand combat but you are going to win.

And at some stage, when you want to get free of your bondage *enough*, the scales will tip and you will decide that *even if it kills you (which it won't) you will refuse the accusing voice.*

A lady that I love dearly shared with me her former experience; she was terrified of going out. I know we are not discussing general fears and phobias here, but she shared this with me to support me when I was bound up. Her fear of going out was huge. But her frustration with that fear was growing too. I believe God was working in her and setting her on the road to freedom. She came to the point of thinking something like this: "Living like this is death. It's not life. It's not abundance. The worst thing that can happen to me if I go outside is that I die. So – not much change from the way I am 'living' then... I'll do it. I'm actually going to do it."

Of course, she went out and the *power of the fear* was broken. As she went, *reality arrived*. It had never really been about inside or outside. There was a spiritual battle going on, and she needed to step into her victory, won for her at the Cross. This lovely lady is now in her seventies, a valued Christian minister who has since travelled with her dear husband both nationally and internationally. *Thank you, Lord Jesus.*

Crisis Moment

I am being absolutely serious here. It's a bit like one of those moments in a movie where a character is utterly convinced they are about to die. Here is the fatal moment. The bomb is about to explode, your eyes are shut, you are simply waiting for the almighty bang when... silence. Nothing happens.

Nothing happens. You hear nothing. You are aware that you are still alive. You hear your watch ticking in the stillness and the sound of your breathing.

I praise God that the fact that you are reading this book is further evidence to you that your release from the tyranny of OCD and accusation is well on the way! Had I not found release, this book would not be in your hands right now. *Jesus, we love you and give you all the glory!*

To the person who believes, or fears, that it would terrible, disastrous, not to check the back door *again*, you are about to discover that the temporary comfort that your repeated checking provides you is, in fact, merely food for the next 'need to check'. But – on the other hand – if you can resist the fear, resist the accusation that you are a careless man or woman who is putting the whole of your family home in jeopardy and probably, also, opening up the whole neighbourhood to a crime wave – if you can move against this tide and *experience* for yourself the *absence of following disaster* – you will learn, first hand, that the pressure to check was a *lie*.

My battle, as I have already begun to share with you, was with a form of OCD called *scrupulosity*. I had to learn that nothing terrible would happen if I wasn't *exactly right* in the way that I communicated with people. A lightning bolt from heaven would not strike me if I moved against accusing thoughts and managed not to obey their demands.

- "Steve, what if you exaggerated when you told Alison about the film? You need to apologise to her and admit you were trying to impress her."

- "Steve, that woman saw the way you looked at her. You need to go apologise for making her feel uncomfortable."

- "Look at that scratch on the wall. *You* did that. You need to own up. Offer to pay for the repair. If you don't, you're guilty."

- "You told the electricity company that you were not available for a meter reading visit next Saturday. That was a lie. You just didn't *want* them to come. You need to contact them and admit you lied…"

The Cross

Can you see that what I was really trying to do was to 'clear myself', 'clean my slate' (whether it needed cleaning or not). In effect, the adversary was tempting me to rely on myself for my right standing with God rather than on the Cross.

I hope I don't even need to say that *of course* it's sensible to lock your car door; it is good to try to right a wrong, if possible, to pick up your litter if you drop it, to apologise to someone if you need to, etc. In the flux of everyday living, sometimes we need to do that. But that is not the kind of reasonable dynamic I am describing here.

My freedom has come with revelation. Revelation has been, and is, central to my recovery.

10

REMEDY: UNDERSTANDING THE OCD SPIKE

Now this chapter really is for those of you struggling with OCD, those of you standing with an OCD-er and those of you who would appreciate being informed and educated!

I found 'the spike' to be a very useful term. I want to link it with some of what I said previously about identifying a spirit of condemnation.

Think of a spike – you could picture a literal spike, you know, a sharp implement of some description. Or you could think of it as a 'wave' which surges to a peak – the wave *spikes* to a maximum potency.

This spike pokes and gives the impression or sensation of piercing. This wave rises in power and threatens to overwhelm.

Let's get something settled here.

The spike is fear – pure and simple. Or maybe we should be more accurate: *impure* and simple.

Let's go with the literal spike for a moment. A sharp discomfort nudges you, prods you; it demands your attention; it demands to be satisfied; it demands to be obeyed.

It says "You must..." It says "If you don't ... it will be your fault; you will be guilty."

The pain of the prodding grows; it comes to a head and you decide to comply with a response that will take the discomfort away. You respond with an action that you believe will remove the spike.

And it does so, *temporarily*. Until the next time, until the next spike arrives either relating to the same issue or to a different one.

> ## Compliance attracts the next spike.

Compliance attracts the next spike.

As one commentator put it, it is like getting into a swimming pool of freezing water. Everything about the situation says you are going to die. "Get out! Get out!" your senses scream. But, actually, if you can just hold on for a few moments, if you can just 'ride' the discomfort and the thoughts which assault your mind, you will see that you are not going to die. You will see that actually the cold water is not going to kill you. In other words, *nothing is really wrong at all*.

Someone else described it as *mind noise*.

The college where I work at has been undergoing significant refurbishment. Over the first day or two, the noise of drilling, hammering and a swathe of other bombarding sounds seemed to have the potential to drive us all bonkers! Several months on, I have to say that the noise became a background feature rather than the *threat* which it had first appeared to be.

When the OCD sufferer gives in to the spike in order to find rest and relief, he is only really empowering it for the next occasion.

By resisting it, he learns that it is a lie. It is unreal. It is a mirage of the mind. Oh, it *appears* to be there, for sure. The *sensation* is certainly there. But the supposed threat is not a real one.

My pastors, along with certain friends, showed me great love, grace and patience as my battles came to a head. They gave me permission to *discover the truth*.

I was so plagued with guilt and fear of being disobedient to God. Accusations assaulted my mind. On one occasion my pastors said to me, "Steve, when these thoughts come, understand that they are not important. And if they really seem to be so, they still aren't."

On another occasion, they gave me permission to "be disobedient" to the Pointing Finger. This was significant. I was being affirmed at a crucial time when I was taking the risk of not responding to a spike.

You often hear Christians talking about "faith, not feelings", but another friend helped me enormously after a long telephone call. We chatted about the nature of the Father, the power of His grace that He had demonstrated at the Cross, and about our new position in Jesus.

"Steve, if it *feels* like OCD, then take it that it is..." is a paraphrase of his advice. I found this, too, tremendously liberating. I was free to reject these accusations. Father knew my heart, knew that I loved Him and that I had given myself to Him as wholly as I knew how. I might make mistakes but His Spirit would not deal with me in the currency of dread and fear, but rather in an affirming fathering which would bring liberty and growth.

11

ID

In my previous book, 'Blood and Glory – The Cross is still the Crux'[7], I referred to a movie, 'The Truman Show', and shared how it impacted me in the area of identity and how the Holy Spirit is working in our lives to *reveal* who we are in Jesus.

Well, here's another one...

Films can be like modern day parables and illustrate human and spiritual dynamics really well. 'ID' is a film made in 1995, written by Jim Bannon and Vincent O'Connell, directed by Philip Davis. I would not particularly recommend that you watch it in that it's a violent, expletive-filled tale of a man's demise into near insanity.

> **Do we know Whose we have become?**

You're probably wondering why I would have even watched such a movie! Well, I was attracted by the title. Then, when I saw that it revolved around a football context, I warmed to the idea. The theme of identity is, I believe, a very important one in the world of Christendom. We are going to stand or fall upon not only who we are in Jesus, but also upon how we see ourselves. Who do you really think you are? Do we know *Whose* we have become and which *Family* we are now part of? (The capital letters in the last two sentences have been added for emphasis, of course!)

---

[7] See Bibliography (p.106)

In 'ID', John is a policeman who is assigned a role in an undercover team of four officers; their task is to infiltrate an east London gang of soccer hooligans, gain valuable insights and information on the pivotal members, with the goal (pardon the pun) of gaining sufficient evidence to lead to arrests and prosecutions.

The department's previous attempts have failed, resulting in a vicious assault on the unfortunate 'outed' police officers. Now, to be successful, John and his colleagues are going to need to be very convincing so as not to arouse the suspicions of the gang members. They are going to have to *live* this role, fully enter into it, embrace it, become it; it's an all or nothing deal. Despite a tentative start from one or two of John's colleagues, especially as they begin to see close up the depths of wanton vandalism and violence which are part and parcel of belonging to the gang, John and the three others manage to become recognised as real football supporters and, more importantly, as *bona fide* hell-raisers.

In between days at football matches and evenings in the gang's regular hangout, a local East End pub, the four officers discuss their progress and consider their next steps. It becomes evident that there is a tension between the perceived need to enter fully into the gang's activities and the need to remain focused on the job in hand. It's not an easy balance to strike, and arguments arise between the four; they are police officers – this is who they are – and yet the developing momentum of their involvement with the gang requires them to tolerate and participate in criminal acts.

You can imagine the irony, I am sure. They are officers who, much of the time as undercover hooligans, are fighting and scheming against the very police force that they are part of.

John is the main character. We see a dramatic change in him as the story develops, and the collapse of his relationship with his girlfriend; she watches with dismay the deterioration in her man's character. A distance emerges between him and his fellow assignees; they seem to have a handle on the requirements of the role whilst at the same time remaining fully aware of who they really are; they are *police officers*. John, however, has an identity problem.

Landing Strips

John appears, at first, to be the stronger, the braver of the four in the team. On one occasion, after a 'meet'[8] is rumbled by the police, one of the original gang members accuses him of being an undercover policeman, which of course he is. Somebody must have 'tipped off' the police, and the gang believe that they have a traitor in their midst. It's a pivotal moment.

John plays the situation beautifully. Whereas an exposed police officer would, in all probability, have betrayed their failure by showing unease and no small measure of fear, John goes on the offensive. He works himself up into a rage, challenging his accuser to a fight outside "right now", breaking a snooker cue in half as his weapon of choice. Witnessing this response, other gang members intervene, protesting John's innocence, which results in his accuser having to stand down and even apologise. John's position, especially, has now strengthened even further.

This is how well John is playing the role. Except, as you may now have gathered, something more sinister is occurring. John appears to be morphing into the very character which, with his colleagues, he was assigned to investigate.

Somewhere in his lack of wholeness as a man, somewhere within this broken psyche, a *landing strip* exists upon which a horde of demons have landed. Now, his inner insecurity feeding on the attention and respect of other group members, he revels in the limelight as being considered one of the 'top boys' in the gang. Any tenderness he had for his girlfriend has vanished; he spurns her and cheats on her; he verbally abuses his colleagues and ever increasingly seeks out violent disorder on the streets.

---

[8] a pre-arranged fight between opposing gangs of football hooligans

This is now an identity crisis in full swing. He seems to have 'found himself', he feels that he belongs in this environment with its kudos and glory, and is painfully unaware of the depths to which he has sunk.

As the film nears its conclusion, the police force decide to abandon the project, dissatisfied with the unsatisfactory results. This comes as a relief to the three colleagues who have seen enough and have come to their wits' end as far as John is concerned. Unsurprisingly, John is furious at this decision.

What has happened here? John's wound, that inner wound where he craved recognition, has now been laid bare. His emptiness is fully exposed. He needs his gang role and involvement. Having so completely given himself to it, he now has nothing left, as his employer insists that the four officers separate themselves completely from the football environment.

The end of the film, whilst perhaps designed to cast some doubt as to whether John really has had a meltdown, suggests to me further confirmation that this desperate man is in dire trouble.

A group of officers are designated to police a 'far right' march; a pack of shaven-headed (mainly young) men stride down the street, shouting Nazi slogans and making fascist salutes. One of John's colleagues makes his way into the throng; he has spotted John, shaven-headed, who is marching with the group. When questioned by his disbelieving colleague, John says that he is on a job and that his cover is in danger of being blown.

I think, by now, the viewer knows better. Our fears appear to be confirmed as the movie comes to a close with a shot of John, saluting and shouting in a frenzy. He wants to belong, he craves the comradeship, his callous heart can only pump on the adrenalin of confrontation and disorder.

His ID is in chaos.

ID

So why have I shared with you this account?

In Christ Jesus, our feet have been planted on a secure, sure foundation. Foundations are meant to be built upon. In Christ we have become sons – royal sons of the King of Kings. I believe that makes you a prince. If you would rather be called a princess, that's fine by me.

You are royalty.

You are royalty.

Our openness to the Holy Spirit is crucial in these days. He really does want to have a close, intimate relationship with us so that He can befriend us, embrace us, heal us, affirm us, fill us with holy power and send us!

He does not force Himself upon us but responds to our invitations. As we live in the Holy Spirit, as we live in union and in partnership with Him, we are going to know a healthy relationship with God. He will teach us, counsel us, reveal mysteries to us and, at times, reveal the roots of those things that have been miseries. The Holy Spirit can open up mysteries and unearth miseries!

It is important that He does this work in our lives so that we do not have unhealed landing strips in our lives upon which the enemy would like to land. We do not want him on our territory; he has nothing we need and has nothing to say that we need to hear. He might have been involved in elements of our past, but he is not going to hold influence in our future! Amen to that!

This close living with the Holy Spirit will shut the door on enemy accusations. Our spirit man will witness with the Holy Spirit and with our true identity in Jesus, and we will be able to swiftly brush off the lying accusations that hell would try to bind us with.

12

LEGITIMATE NEEDS

It's fine that we have needs.

> "With intimate knowing, He understands what excites us and what we are passionate about. He knows the depths of our longings and our greatest dreams. He knows why we are passionate and how this zeal is a glorious part of who He made us to be."[9]

We were created to be in relationship with God, first and foremost. The Bible says that He made everything (including us) and that in Him all things hold together. Removing Him from the equation would be like expecting a bicycle wheel to function normally having removed the centre spindle to which the spokes are attached.

We were created to live in relationship with others. We are social beings by design. As we interact with each other healthily and positively, we blossom and grow and are able to express our uniqueness and who we really are.

Jesus said that He had come to give us *abundant* life. That's a definition of overflowing, splashing *life!* We were not made to simply exist, to breathe God's air and fill our stomachs. Life has a vibrancy when God is the senior partner in its journey.

In his book, 'The Seven Longings of the Human Heart', Mike Bickle identifies and highlights some of the key needs with which we were

[9] Mike Bickle; see Bibliography (p.106)

created. Secular theorists such as Maslow are well known for their conclusions concerning not only physical needs such as water, warmth and shelter, but also higher needs such as significance and belonging. You may wish to use a search engine to check out Maslow's triangular hierarchy of needs.

Mike Bickle shared that we long to be enjoyed by our God and that He has made us not to *wander* aimlessly but to *wonder.* We love to be fascinated, to be captivated, don't we? We long for intimacy and to be surrounded by, and live amid, beauty. He shares that there is nothing wrong with expecting greatness from our lives; a mighty, great, all loving God created us, and He created us to demonstrate His greatness! It's good that we want to make an impact on our world and to be wholehearted about our mission as Christ's ambassadors.

Nevertheless, most of us have not been raised in a perfect environment where each and every influence ushered us towards such goals.

Needy People

The truth is that we have all been influenced, to one degree or another, by needy people, by those who perhaps have not had lives centred in Jesus.

Some of us have been tolerated rather than embraced. Some have rarely been touched. Some have been touched in a wrong way, maybe sexually or violently. Some were raised with little or no affirmation, or with a continual eye of criticism lingering over their progress. Some have not been allowed to *breathe* and become who they truly are. Some have found themselves to be square pegs in round holes as influential personalities around them have imposed their wills upon them.

Some came to Christ with a good deal of baggage. We have become accustomed to its weight, its feel, its features. Some have as good as accepted that this load is actually part of who they are, rather than an unwelcome addition which has kept them company for so long. Some have accepted the barbed words of others as truth and clothed themselves with them: "You will never be able to…" "You always /

never..." "Everybody thinks you're..."; "You're a waste of space / stupid / fat / ugly..." and so on.

It is no wonder that many of our churches resemble hospitals as much as spiritual army units.

And I think that's fine, actually, as long as each of us are open to the Holy Spirit's work in us. He wants to heal us, restore, affirm, re-invigorate. As He is free to work with us we become more open to the moving of the Holy Spirit in our lives; He reveals aspects of Himself to us and touches our hunger – kindles that sense of fascination I mentioned a moment ago. We become able to look away from ourselves and increasingly to the needy around us. In so doing, the Holy Spirit sparks into life some of those traits and qualities we have been gifted with. As we do so, we are investing in lives and in the lives of those our contacts will meet. Do you see that? I can represent Christ to people around me in certain ways because others *invested in me*, they took time to be a part of my healing and restoration, and others will do so in the future. Thanks to them, people I meet now will not be subject to facets of the unhealed Steve of yesteryear.

Each piece of work that the Holy Spirit does in us is precious. It is permanent; it works; it is an excellent job! It reduces the possibility that the enemy will be able to hoodwink us, deceive us and waylay us into walking in the flesh and in wrong identity. Our vulnerability to being enticed, seduced and accused by him lessen with each dealing of the Holy Spirit in our lives.

Discipline

And – we need discipline, right? We need those around us who will care enough to set us straight sometimes.

There's a huge difference between being motivated by the Holy Spirit to bring correction to someone, and criticising them from a hard or insecure heart.

The Pointing Finger

If I am jealous of you, the quickest way I can get us to the same level is to pull you down to mine. Sound familiar?

13

UNDERMINING – SOCIETY'S PASTIME

Apparently we are very good at doing this in the UK.

Part of this impression may stem from the well-known dry British sense of humour. I have to admit I tend to have such a sense of humour myself. Others may disagree but I think that sarcasm, though considered to be the 'lowest form of wit' by some commentators, can be very funny indeed as long as the motive is not to genuinely belittle another; between good friends it can provide a lot of hilarity. Sarcastic remarks are often ironic in nature but cross the line, in my opinion, if there is an intent to wound someone in any respect.

———————

A man died and went to heaven. As he stood at the Pearly Gates, he saw a huge wall of clocks behind him. He asked, "What are all those clocks?"

The angel, with clipboard, answered, "Those are sarcasm-clocks. Everyone on Earth has a sarcasm-clock. Every time you're sarcastic the hands on your clock will move."

"Oh right," said the man, "and I suppose that *really* happens… NOT!"

"That's Mother Teresa's," continued the angel. "The hands have never moved, indicating that she never berated anyone with sarcasm."

"Incredible," said the man.

"That's Abraham Lincoln's clock. The hands have moved seven times, telling us that Abe yielded to sarcasm just seven times in his entire life."

"Where's my clock?" asked the man.

"Oh, your clock is in Jesus' office. He's using it as a fan."

I am not sure where the more official evidence for the view of the British comes from. I imagine that much of it is anecdotal although I have heard several references to the sense of humour of Londoners which helped them to stick together and make it through the Second World War.

> ...we smugly respond, "I told you so."

But, we do seem to be quite good at building people up and then undermining them until they fall. Then we smugly respond, "I told you so."

It could be a politician. It could be a sports personality. The media hype clamours for a certain individual to be installed in a position, elevated, and then, once they are there, almost appears to hope for their failure.

Capello – A Case in Point

When Fabio Capello was touted as becoming the new manager of the England football team (a very significant role for a nation so enamoured with its sport – especially football!) hopes of success and development of the game soared! This successful Italian was going to be the answer to our success-starved prayers.

He wasn't like your typical English football manager. This guy exuded class, was very polite and softly spoken (although initially his English was weak) and inflated the British ego as we revelled in the possibility of being led by a man of such calibre.

Pride began to rise, hopes ascended rapidly to notions of international silverware.

This was *the* Fabio Capello; he was an Italian, a devout Catholic who was interested in fine art. *He had won the domestic league title of every club he had managed.* Happy days were coming to English football. The nation rejoiced too at the prospect of overpaid footballers coming under the wing of a disciplined coach, one known to exact a stricter regime than former England managers, who had seemed to be over-lenient on occasions.

Results in 2008, after Capello's appointment, were very good – five wins in the first six games. England went on to qualify easily for the 2010 World Cup. However, two draws were followed by a narrow 1-0 victory over Slovenia, which raised eyebrows but nevertheless saw the team qualify for the knockout stages of the competition.

Well, there's nothing like a game against our old rivals, Germany, to inspire passions!

England were outclassed and lost 4-1. The manner of the defeat demonstrated the gulf in class between the nations, and questions surfaced as to whether the team and, more widely, English football had really developed at all.

Tales then emerged concerning Capello's disciplined regime during the tournament. What had been perceived as a strength was now reported as a weakness: he had been overbearing; senior players had not been permitted to have input.

Whether this had been true or not, it was interesting to witness the swing in the nation's attitude to Capello. The press had gone from hot to cold. Capello used outdated tactics, it was now claimed; his selection of certain players had been suspect. Although he stayed on to see England qualify for their next major tournament, he resigned following the Football Association's involvement concerning his choice of England team captain.

Newspaper headlines ridiculing Capello included:

"PRAT IN A HAT"

...alongside a photo of the manager during a goalless draw with Montenegro.

"FOOL MONTE"

...relating to the same game.

"JACKASS"

...declared a tabloid, showing a photo of Capello with superimposed donkey's ears.

Negative Air

This suggests to me a rather desperate corporate insecurity. *You* fail, we can huddle together with pointing fingers, and then no-one will be examining *me*. This attitude, this mentality surrounds us. But it is not a Kingdom quality.

Of course, though we are seated in heavenly places in the Kingdom of God, we reside within earthly bodies on a fallen planet. The "prince of the power of the air"[10], as our adversary is named, fills the air with negative, Christ-less propaganda. And if he knows that you and I have seen him for what and who is he, he can only try to distract and bewitch us with doubt and accusation, to tempt us to walk out from under the identity umbrella which covers us and not only accuse ourselves but also others.

Covered

It's a red umbrella, coated in the Blood of Jesus which saved us and transferred our ownership. Whereas an umbrella generally is used to keep the rain off you, this umbrella has rain falling upon you from

---

[10] Ephesians 2:2

within it, from inside it. You and I, in Christ, walk under a waterfall of grace, as Pastor Joseph Prince describes it.

You've heard, I'm sure, of the 'clean as you go' approach to hygiene, particularly within commercial (and especially food) environments. I used to work at a well-known pizza chain, and that was certainly the policy.

Well, the Blood of Jesus cleansed us once for all at the Cross – we are clean as we go. That is our position. We may slip up from time to time but our state remains the same. Recognising this kindness of the Lord towards us is what produces true repentance in us (Romans 2:4). That has certainly been my own experience.

I want to look now at a very common arena of enemy accusation.

14

WRONG RESPONSIBILITY

This is an area of accusation that I have walked through and seen close up. It's very prevalent, and I think that it goes unnoticed a lot of the time. People often don't realise that they are responding through a lens of wrong responsibility.

PROVERBS 29:25

"The fear of man brings a snare,
But he who trusts in the LORD will be exalted."

I like the first part of The Message's rendering which says:

PROVERBS 29:25 (THE MESSAGE)

"The fear of human opinion disables…"

According to this word, the fear of man has the very opposite effect to that which we would like to achieve! We usually alter our actions or reactions in an attempt to assuage fear or placate someone who may cause us anxiety. It's a response of self-protection.

But the Bible says that it is the Lord who exalts us – He lifts us above the situation – as we place out trust in Him, not in ourselves. We disable ourselves, hindering ourselves and our goals, as we try to please someone because of fear.

It's great to want to please others; generous hearts do that! But that is a completely different dynamic to the one which I am describing where there is not freedom but a bondage to fear.

Julie has had a phone call from her sister, Tammy. "She's going to be in town over the weekend and needs somewhere to stay. I'd normally offer her our spare bedroom, but John and I were really looking forward to a nice, quiet weekend together; it's been rough since John lost his job and we just need some 'down time'. But I can't possibly say no – what would she think? She'd be so offended... No, it's much easier all round just to let her come."

Do you recognise a scenario like this?

Generous people give of themselves. They want to please others, bless others. They are prepared to put others' wishes above their own. But this is not healthy if it is at the expense of the Spirit life, at the expense of right order.

If I prefer you because I want to bless you, and in so doing I am blessed, that's one thing. It is certainly a delight to give and to do so extravagantly. But if I prefer you because I am afraid to say no, I reveal a different motivation, and *the fruit will be equally different*. If the source of my action is one of bondage, then that's the kind of fruit my action will yield even though it appears that I am being generous and that I am acceding to your request.

In our scenario above, Julie needs to say, "Not this time, sweetie." When we walk in the fear of the

Truth works in the light.

Lord (preferring Him above others) we walk in *peace*. And, even though her sister might not get what she wants, Julie's stance would bring light into their relationship. Truth works in the light.

Julie does not need to explain herself, justify herself, tell her sister *why* the answer is no. It's no and that's it.

The Privilege of Relationship

If you and I are in relationship, that is a privilege for us both. It's something to be grateful for, to enjoy, to guard and to respect. To whatever degree that relationship is, you and I have granted each other a measure of space and influence in each other's life. We have given each other *permission* to interact at a certain, mutually agreed level of intimacy.

If our level of intimacy is such that you have permission to ask me to do something then I, equally, have permission to say yes or no without explanation. You and I may volunteer those reasons but we are under no obligation whatsoever to provide them. If I feel that I am *under obligation* to tell you why, it may be because there is an undercurrent of fear or manipulation in the relationship. *I* am actually trying to convince *you* that I am making the correct decision. But you don't need to know if it is the right decision or not. You just need to know my decision. Because it *is* the right decision for me.

Do you see that if it is the *wrong* decision for me then, in truth, it is also the wrong decision for you? Something about our relationship needs to be brought into the light; I am hiding from you my true feelings on the issue and allowing your will to be imposed on it over mine.

Julie's time is hers to *give*. If, by the Holy Spirit, she senses a prompting to yield that time – or she simply wants to do so – all well and good. In the scenario I set out, she wants to spend time with John; that is the right thing to do in her view so she really needs to stand by her conviction.

Please understand I am not trying to suggest that we stop blessing people! But blessers are also blessed; if I apparently bless you and in doing so lose my peace and sense of blessing, "something ain't right", as they say around these parts!

"Sorry Tammy, that weekend doesn't work for me... Perhaps we could..."

Manipulation

Watch out for those manipulative voices. You'll know their source from the fruit they birth in you. Do you sense an excitement with a particular suggestion or a heavy weight or dread?

I really do not like to be manipulated! It offends my spirit too. I think, "How dare you try to usurp authority!"

"I just don't know *how* I'm going to get to the shops in time before my appointment later. Oh dear, what am I going to do?"

Stop it! If you would like a lift to the shops, *ask me for one*. But please don't whine and play the victim card. It betrays a lack of character. Ask me for a lift – you may well have 'permission' within our relationship to do that. And I will exercise my freedom too to say yes or no. Simple.

It can happen in church scenarios too. Again, please hear me. Let's do anything to bless each other, and none of us are beyond helping to put the chairs out, making tea and coffee, greeting on the door and scrubbing the toilets. So you preach and prophesy? Amen and great. How about washing up next Sunday?

On the other hand, no-one has the right to push you into a commitment which simply does not witness with your spirit.

"We really feel that you should be part of the intercessory team and attend the meeting on Wednesday evenings."

All right, thank you, that might be exciting. I'm going to think on that for a few days because, to be honest, it doesn't immediately resound inside of me. I'm a sheep and I hear His voice, so I'll let you know.

You see, the Holy Spirit might show you or me that this absolutely is something He wants to nurture and grow in our life. Or, the notion might stay as flat as a pancake for you, and you just sense, "This is not for me – at least, not for now."

We need to go with our conviction. Our "Yes" is yes and our "No" is no.

15

GOD, OUR SHIELD AND DEFENDER

It is amazing the lengths we go to, sometimes, to defend ourselves, when God has said that defending us is His job.

I have a lot to learn in this area but I have seen the Lord do wonderful work in people around me who are catching on far quicker than I am.

I remember a wonderful testimony from John Bevere[11] in this vein. I will not go into all the details here, but the bare bones of it are that he had, at one time, a difficult relationship with a person in authority in his church circle. John was unfairly accused in some respect and he wanted to right the situation. It was quite a struggle for him, understandably. He wanted to defend himself. You and I would probably feel very similar. The issue was serious enough to threaten to cause him to resign a ministry position.

He prayed about it, of course, and subsequently some evidence came across his path of wrongdoing on the part of his accuser. At first sight, this appeared to be the Lord's intervention and means of vindicating John. Praise God, He had answered! From what I remember it wasn't that John wanted to get even; he just wanted to clear his name and re-balance the situation. However, an unease settled upon our man of God, and he sensed that the Lord was showing him that *it was not his place to uncover this other leader*. It's challenging, isn't it?

---

[11] See Bibliography (p.107)

In fact, John only had peace on this issue when he decided to obey the Holy Spirit and *destroy the evidence* concerning his accuser which was in his possession. That cannot have been easy but if you, like me, have sensed the Lord's weighty hand upon you concerning a matter, it's better to yield!

John was obedient. I do not remember the timescales involved, exactly, but a while later, while John was away, out of the area, further evidence of wrongdoing surfaced concerning this church leader, and he was removed from his position. John was vindicated and *he wasn't even in town.*

PSALM 7:8

"Let the Lord judge the peoples. Vindicate me, Lord, according to my righteousness, according to my integrity, O Most High."

In the New International Version, Psalm 57:1-3 says:

"Have mercy on me, my God, have mercy on me,
    for in you I take refuge.
I will take refuge in the shadow of your wings
    until the disaster has passed.
I cry out to God Most High,
    to God, who vindicates me.
He sends from heaven and saves me,
    rebuking those who hotly pursue me.
God sends forth his love and his faithfulness."

John Bevere did well. He cried out to the Lord, not to others! God 'sent from heaven' and 'rebuked his pursuer' in His love and His faithfulness.

I am rather too quick to defend myself on occasions. I suppose I justify it in the name of pursuing truth and justice. I am not saying that it is always appropriate to remain silent on an issue; we need to be led by Holy Spirit in all things and it might be right to speak up. The issue, though, is still relevant, as I know that my *real* motive for defending myself may not be as noble as I may try to suggest. The deal for me to consider is, am I going to trust God or not? Am I going to try to take matters into my own

> **...am I going to trust God or not?**

hands or to trust the favour of the Lord to come through for me? Am I prepared to wait for Him to do that, even if it means that, for a time, my name is being spoken of negatively, *even* in the public domain?

When we have the fear of the Lord, we will be able to exercise some wisdom concerning our response to the accusations of others. I love the fact that certain authors and speakers who have been (and still are) publicly criticised and even slandered actually include these comments on their own websites! That's what I call standing up to the accuser!

Isaiah prophesied:

ISAIAH 53:7

"He was oppressed and He was afflicted,
Yet He did not open His mouth;
Like a lamb that is led to slaughter,
And like a sheep that is silent before its shearers,
So He did not open His mouth."

In the Living Bible, the verse reads:

ISAIAH 53:7 (TLB)

"He was oppressed and he was afflicted, yet he never said a word. He was brought as a lamb to the slaughter; and as a sheep before her shearers is dumb, so he stood silent before the ones condemning him."

If anyone *ever* had the right (as we understand it) to defend His innocence, it was Jesus of Nazareth. Not only did he not do so, but He appeared to allow his enemies to win the argument completely, even to going to the Cross.

On the Cross the accusations and taunts continued:

MATTHEW 27:40

"You who are going to destroy the temple and rebuild it in three days, save Yourself! If You are the Son of God, come down from the cross."

The New Living Translation offers the first part of the verse as:

MATTHEW 27:40A (TLB)

"'Look at you now!' they yelled at him..."

Isn't it amazing that we get to partner with Jesus in the vindication! You see, Jesus followed through on His mission – His love fuelled Him to do that. Because He completed the mission, there are now millions of people filled with the Holy Spirit, learning to exercise Kingdom authority on the earth. We are walking, talking evidence of Jesus' ministry. He is vindicated through our love for Him and influence on the earth.

16

ADDICTION: MY NAME IS STEVE…

…and I'm an alcoholic.

So goes the well versed opening statement for those introducing themselves at Alcoholics Anonymous. (I am not an alcoholic, by the way.)

The round of applause which greets the brave admission is well deserved; it's certainly a start to bringing issues into the light and establishing some accountability. However, we still need the *power* to overcome those issues, not only to stop certain behaviours or even to get into the habit of replacing them with more healthy alternatives, but to *become changed.*

In Christ we have become a new creation, right? The old has gone and the new has come.

Look, I want to encourage you. I know this isn't the condition-specific manual or self-help guide that you can surely find elsewhere, and I expect you'll have a wide choice to choose from. But I can tell you that Jesus Christ is the power in you to free you from your addictions.

> **Religion will not do it.**

Religion will not do it. But the living God is able. And He knows the real you better than you know yourself. I wonder if you are willing to let him take the reins and work with you.

Addiction

Dare you admit – is 'recognise' a friendlier word than 'admit'? – dare you *recognise* that addiction is a form of bondage in your life?

I love the way that David Wong puts it when he compares the nature of *addiction* to that of *enjoyment*.

> "There's a distinct difference between simply enjoying a thing versus having a compulsion to do it. It's 'want' versus 'need'. I like wearing jeans, for instance. I would wear them every day if allowed. But when my workplace banned them and I went three straight years without wearing a single pair, the lack of jeans didn't cause me anxiety. I didn't sit there at my desk and fidget and have to constantly turn my mind away from my jeanlessness. I didn't have to constantly stop myself from reaching for them in my closet.
>
> Compare that to 'John', who had to be virtually restrained in a straightjacket when he tried to quit smoking. Or compare that to the guy who loses $20,000 at the blackjack table and has to sell his children on the Thai sex market to pay off gambling debts. That's addiction. When you come back and do something again and again because your brain has got hooked into thinking you have to, everything else be damned."[12]

Sometimes it's not an easy call as to whether there is an addictive pattern.

Maggie drinks coffee every morning after she gets up. If she misses her super skinny latte she has a sinking feeling before half past ten. Is she just thirsty? Is it just a habit? We like our habits. We choose to have that super skinny (or whatever yours is) because we like the taste, right?

Or, maybe it started that way but, actually, now there is something else going on too. Our senses, our body – it feels like my *whole system*

---

[12] www.cracked.com; see Bibliography (p.106)

needs that drink to get my day going. I'm not talking about the natural need for water for the purposes of hydration, or calories for some early 'get up and go', am I? You can tell the difference.

Perhaps it's not the coffee – for you. Perhaps it's a cigarette. Perhaps it used to be a cigarette but now it's three cigarettes. Perhaps it used to be three standard cigarettes but now it's a stronger variety. Or marijuana. The smell from that is especially awkward so you have managed to convince your colleagues at the office that you adore extra strong mints; there's always a packet of them on your desk.

Perhaps you end the day and start the next one with a dose of pornography. Is it that you *enjoy* looking at it, or is it that you think you *need* to do so? As David Wong says, the absence of indulging the habit produces anxiety. If, for some reason, you do not manage to view this material, you actually feel frustrated – even angry. You may have told your spouse that you are struggling in this area, but you may well not have. Is that because you feel it is *under control?* Are you *under its control?* Is the habit controlling you by convincing you that you can keep it a secret?

Perhaps you are ministering next Sunday and intersperse your preparation with pornographic episodes.

Jesus has something much better for us.

There are, of course, the more respectable addictions such as shopping, television, computer games and sports. Keeping fit seems to be a major one. There's nothing wrong with keeping fit, of course, but when that drive to exercise becomes obsessional, when someone *needs* the adrenalin fix, we are in different territory.

Please understand, too, that I am not speaking against committed goal seeking and achieving – the businessman who wants to succeed and excel, the athlete who wants to win his crown, or the pastor who wants to see his church move on in God and impact his locality.

The issue is, *what is behind the drive?* Is the drive in its place as a servant, or is it becoming a master?

Pete enjoys going to the gym. He recognised that he needed to lose some weight and enrolled at his local sports centre. He's married with two children, works in the city and only has one evening he can commit to his new health focus. From time to time he is unable to make it to his training session – life happens, doesn't it? – other calls on his time arise. He would have preferred to go to the gym but... fine. *There is no inner discomfort* at his missing his session.

Carolina's interest in the game of chess began when she was a teenager. She found it to be more inspiring than some of the more common, regular pursuits of many of her peers. Her interest in the hobby fluctuated until her best friend bought her a chess computer. It really was a beautiful, thoughtful gift. This self-contained unit was more user friendly than many of the online programs and computer software that Carolina had dabbled with previously, and she quickly embarked upon a campaign of competition with the machine. And there was a lot of competition to be had: Chess Emperor came with eighteen built-in levels, along with 'tutorial mode' help and mini sessions where particular moves and strategies could be explored.

Hmm... *explored*. We need to come back to that word.

You know where this is going, right? Her time spent on Chess Emperor increased as she battled for mastery. It was almost as if the machine was programmed to allow her to get so far, so close to victory, she would think that her winning move was imminent until – *slam!* Her hardy opponent, seemingly from nowhere, would make what, in itself, appeared to be an insignificant move, and Carolina would find herself on the back foot, facing defeat once again.

Not that she hadn't made progress. As a level ten player she was no newbie any longer. But her time with Chess Emperor began to take its toll: on occasions she missed meals; she would become even a little dehydrated during her extensive chess sessions; she cancelled her pottery and dance classes; and two of her mates, whom she used to see fairly regularly, began to wonder why she had stopped contacting them.

She went to sleep in the early hours of the morning with a headache and awoke with one. "Level 11, level 11, level 11..." If she could just get to level 11 – now *that* would be a good level to take a break. Sure, she had thought the same when she was on level 9 and wanted to get to level 10, but *this time* she really would stop after level 11.

This is the mantra of addiction and you may, like me, have heard it: *"Just one more..."*

Just One More

Every addict can relate to the 'Just One More' syndrome, one which hides the lie that the addict is still in control of their compulsive habit. Whether it relates to placing a 'final' bet (oh yes, of course, the very last one...) on the horses, one last drink of pornographic material online or whatever field the addiction operates in, the yielding to 'just one more' is the very evidence that victory has not yet been attained.

Addiction is about something deep inside. We may think that it is the poor who are more likely to succumb to a betting cycle of destruction, but it isn't necessarily the case. The well-off may not need the money, but they often need the buzz, the excitement, the sense of anticipation that induces a euphoric rush when victory is achieved.

And it seems to be so easy! A £5 bet returns £10 – for what? For nothing! For absolutely no work whatsoever. The temptation to up the stakes is not far away. If you can be tempted with a mere morsel then you have potential to be ransacked of all that you own.

Online access has dramatically increased the number of prisoners held in addiction's jails. It's just too easy, isn't it? Offers of 'free', no-loss, introductory bets entice the naive into the net.

Boredom propels people to seek something more. No wonder, too, for God made us to 'buzz' with life, to feel alive and to know the wonder of our senses. But He designed us to find that fulfilment through Him, not outside Him.

With one's feet in the mesh of the net, it doesn't take long before you can't seem to get out. Fear, that common trait of the enemy's kingdom, drives you to raise the stakes; if you can just get one big win, your problems are over. It's a familiar but tragic chat up line.

There will probably be the occasional win, just often enough to maintain the illusion.

Not only is this typical of betting activity but, of course, it is its very design. No one would be stupid enough to bet if winning was an impossibility, and companies wouldn't operate if you were likely to win frequently. Sometimes punters lose in the cruellest ways, for example, betting on a star tennis player to defeat a lesser opponent and yet losing the bet as the star injures him or herself during the match and has to forfeit. You would never have expected that to happen and would never have taken such a possibility into account. Checking any number of form guides or performance reviews would not have covered that eventuality.

I remember an occasion when I placed a bet on a certain football match. It was one of these (now common) in-play wagers, where you simply (oh, so simply) enter the betting game during the sporting event. I placed my bet on two teams drawing their game; there were only five minutes remaining, with the scores level, when I clicked the button.

Two minutes later, one of the teams scored. Boom. Goodbye.

Individuals suffer, families suffer. Marriages break up and houses are sold. The man or woman who apparently 'had everything' is left with nothing but a few bin bags of personal belongings.

Compulsion

Addiction is compulsion. And behind it there is a (sometimes subtle) accusation: "You have not done enough." Coupled with the memory of earlier victories, and even the occasional current win, it's a potent mix.

Addiction is compulsion.

There is nothing wrong with enjoying a game of chess, if that's your thing. I've told you that I enjoy a game of chess and I used to have a chess computer... But it took me down some of the same alleys as Carolina.

Just one more... As if I am in control. As if I am making a clear, firm decision. I have chosen "just one more". *I am deceiving myself.*

"I'll stop. I know I can stop. Just one more. One more drink, one final visit to that pornographic website, one final visit to that swingers club, one final booze cruise, just one more early Sunday morning fishing trip... I know I said that last week's was the last, but this week *really will be...*"

With addiction, it's a self-fulfilling prophecy. It's just that the last one isn't *this* one, it's the one which will follow. When we say "last one", we mean "there will be a next one".

The common thread

We see the common thread that links the themes of this book together:

Addiction says, "Just one more, go on."

Compulsion says, "You just *have* to do this."

Accusation says, "Look what you did!" or "If you don't do this, it'll be your fault."

> **The pointing finger ... makes demands upon us and is never satisfied.**

Pressure. Not peace. The pointing finger that makes demands upon us and is never satisfied. *We have never done enough.*

In Jesus our position is exactly opposite to these manipulative assaults. In Jesus, *He* did enough, and having been placed *in Christ*, there are no outstanding debts to be paid. We are freed to enjoy life without being mastered by it.

17

LET'S GET PHYSICAL!

Attention and priority is rightly given to our spirit man. This is where we live from. This is where we have been knitted to Jesus by the Holy Spirit – we have come home.

There is also a sea of teaching around our *soul;* our make-up, our minds and emotions serve us best when submitted to our spirit man. Our spirit man is always in perfect unity with heaven and heaven's agenda for us, although of course we are on a learning curve in terms of living this out effectively. Our soul, however, needs some re-training and discipline, and there are old habits and ways of thinking to shed and new ones to embrace and embed.

This does not make our physical body unimportant. It is an area that the world and its wisdom gives spectacular attention to. Because the world gives it such prominence does not mean that we are to give it none at all. Our bodies are important; they were fashioned by God and they are going to carry us around for some time! Just because we are born again does not mean that we can afford to neglect our physical health or, dare I say it, our appearance. Ambassadors need to reside and move in well maintained accommodation! Nevertheless, the adversary's accusations also include our physicality so it's worth some consideration here.

Firstly, our inherited nature is bent towards self-criticism. "My hair is too curly." "My legs are too short." "My nose is not absolutely straight." "My breasts are too large." "I don't like my chin." "My eyes..." And so on.

Now, we have the perfect right to air our opinions about our bodies – to ourselves at least, if not publicly, as we so choose! I mean, we do spend rather a significant time in them, don't we?

When I was a pre-teen child, I was comparatively small. Most of the lads in my school class were taller than me. Coupled with the fact that my voice broke a little later than the majority of my peers', you can imagine I had some concentrated ribbing from them at times. Even one of my class teachers called me a Bee Gee! Around the age of fifteen to sixteen, I suddenly shot up! I was quite lanky – sometimes I think I could do with some of that lankiness now because my middle has been expanding a little!

I like my forearms; they are thick set and strong, principally because I have played some squash over the years. I am told I have a nice smile and smiley eyes. But I would prefer to have a manlier chest! However, it would take hours of committed exercise – and, who knows, surgery?! – to manifestly change my build. I have the build I was given and my body (and, I imagine yours, too) defaults to certain parameters – parameters which I believe God set:

PSALM 139:13-14

"For You formed my inward parts;
You wove me in my mother's womb.
I will give thanks to You, for I am fearfully and wonderfully made…"

The New Century Version puts it like this:

PSALM 139:13-14 (NCV)

"You made my whole being;
you formed me in my mother's body.
I praise you because you made me in an amazing and wonderful way.
What you have done is wonderful.
I know this very well."

The enemy can accuse us concerning our bodies, and we need to reject these insinuations and suggestions – most of which are designed to cause us to compare ourselves with others, or with *exemplar* type appearances pushed by the media, or to treat ourselves harshly in some fashion in an attempt to change the way we are.

The fashion and health industries are big business. They exist to make money, probably to make a *few* people *very* rich. If I were to describe the steps required to brush photoshop a model's image, I would probably need more than ten of them.

The health industry, too, is a multi-million dollar business. I have lost count of the contradicting 'evidence' and advice given concerning diet and exercise. I recently watched a documentary which revealed that one of the reasons people with a Body Mass Index (BMI) of 25-30 are termed as overweight is to draw as many people to health products as possible! Did you know that certain tabloid newspaper journalists do deals with celebrities who agree, for a payment, to vary their weight during the year to provide articles for popular magazines?

I am not saying that health is unimportant! Far from it, we need to eat a steady, regular, balanced diet; but I think as long as we get a reasonable amount of exercise too, a few sweet treats along the way are there to be enjoyed!

To What Cost?

I am thinking now of one of my favourite British actresses. I will not give her name. I have enjoyed watching her on television, and I thought she had a lovely smile (as well as a nice voice.) Well, I was very surprised to catch her in a different programme, in a new role and – most surprisingly – with a new appearance! She had undergone facial surgery. I can only imagine the goal was to increase the prominence of her mouth. She has certainly succeeded in her goal. I would suggest that the jury is out on whether it has spoiled or improved her appearance.

But there you go. *I* am making a judgement, aren't I? I guess if *she* is happy with her new look… but don't you think that *generally* we have the bodies we were designed to have? And, as I have said, short of eating properly, keeping reasonably fit and taking some care with our appearance, we probably do best to accept God's design of us.

I mean, there's only one of you and only one of me.

There's only one of you…

I hear there were days (probably before my time!) when it was considered virtuous to dress unattractively and to make no effort with one's appearance – I am thinking here of the ladies especially. I am glad we have largely come out of that way of thinking – nonsense, I would say! I hope that you feel fine about 'dressing to kill' if you want to. But not dressing to *thrill* – now that is a different matter.

We are in this world but not of it. The media, through advertising, daily tries to persuade you that you are dissatisfied.

Guys, grow some muscles, dye your hair, change your car, and immediately attract 75% of the neighbourhood's females with two sprays of Jungle Scent under each armpit!

Ladies, lose several kilos, use special cream which will surely make you look twenty five when you are fifty, buy a sexy little bright red or green runabout, and buy these ready meals which are so convincing in their home-cooked appearance that your friends and family will be awe-inspired and hold you with reverent veneration.

The underlying message seems to be, "You need to be different." And yet, in an apparent contradiction, the message is also, "You need to look like *this* because *this* is what attractive is."

By all means, buy a special watch if you want to, drink a certain liqueur if you enjoy it, upgrade your car, hairstyle and whatever else. That's not the principal point, is it?

This is all fine as long as we can afford it, as long as we are not responding to an accusation that we are currently inadequate in some way, and as long as we are not being mastered by these 'things'.

Real Health

You and I know, don't we, that healthy eating and fitness are common sense. We don't really need to buy a book to tell us that. I am not suggesting that these books and DVDs are a con; I think that they have their place, but I think it fair to say that most medical commentators accept that if we...

- eat a proper, balanced diet;

- exercise reasonably and regularly;

- make friends and avoid isolation;

- enjoy a sense of purpose in our lives...

...then we are likely to keep ourselves in good health. I would add, maybe not unexpectedly, that having a clear purpose to our lives is incomplete without Jesus Christ. In Him, all things hold together.

Here's an encouraging thought: a nurse recently told me that, technically, you could describe half of one of the world's leading rugby teams as obese! We need to be wise to the pressure messages emanating from the media.

Don't be surprised if there is some accusation hidden within some of those enticing, special, 'become the real you' offers!

18

SATISFACTION SOLUTION

Our freedom from accusation (including OCD) and addictions is going to be rooted in both what we *believe* (be-live) about God and ourselves and *our real experience* of Him.

Addictions are like a glass of salt water. We may be so thirsty – so thirsty for love and for life satisfaction – that we will drink almost anything, *even* if we know that there are going to be negative consequences from doing so. Because the moment of thrill, as brief as it is, injects us with an experience. A powerful experience.

If we believe that the salt water is the only variety available, we are doomed to walking in a vicious circle. The very water that we drink causes the thirst which will necessitate the next drink. That is, until we taste the real thing: fresh, cool water.

Coca Cola – that delicious yet sugar-laden soft drink! – did well with one of their famous advertising campaigns. "Coca Cola – the Real Thing", a slogan launched in 1969, served the company well to counter rivals who produced their own colas, hoping for a sniff of the market. You have to say they have been extremely successful, recently marking up a market share (of all carbonated soft drinks) of 42%. That's huge. Their nearest rival, Pepsi, came in at 31%. Of the $35 billion raked in by the company, some $2 billion was spent on advertising. Coca Cola have upgraded their logo at least ten times since starting production in 1896.[13]

In John 10:10, Jesus says:

JOHN 10:10 (AMP)

"The thief comes only in order to steal and kill and destroy. I came that they may have and enjoy life, and have it in abundance (to the full, till it overflows)."

Jesus is the real thing.

Jesus is *the real thing*. He warned us that many would come after Him, claiming to be the real thing (Matthew 24:5). He says that He, Himself, is the giver of overflowing life. Millions of us walking the four corners of the earth in the power of the Holy Spirit, overflowing that life to those around us, would certainly impact the world.

The Holy Spirit wants to revive, energise and impact the church so that we can do the same as Jesus in the world. He is drawing those who are willing into a deep intimacy with Himself because those who *know* Him will be strong (in Him) and achieve much for the Kingdom (Daniel 11:32).

Fraud

Fraud experts tell us that the best way to identify a fake document – a bank note or a passport, for example – is to thoroughly *know* the real things![14]

These trained connoisseurs use their senses of sight and touch to pick out items which masquerade as originals. The Bank of England have produced an online guide to help the public do the same.

In the 2002 movie, 'Catch Me If You Can', directed by Steven Spielberg, a portrayal of the tricks and antics of real-life Frank

---

[13] www.businessinsider.com; see Bibliography (p.106)
[14] www.bankofengland.co.uk; see Bibliography (p.106)

Abagnale Jr in the sixties and seventies, we eventually discover that the most qualified police expert is... Abagnale himself. In a deal with the police, he agrees to help the Fraud Squad solve the insolvable cases in return for a monitored freedom outside jail. Who better to advise and support the police than an ex-con whose skills and even instinct for detecting the fake amongst the real cannot be bettered?

We have been deeply influenced by the fake, but by spending time with, and getting to know, Father, Son and Holy Spirit, we will become qualified discerners of the truth.

The easiest way to evangelise is to live Life. Life with Jesus, in Him and through Him. It's not an act; just being yourself in the power of the Holy Spirit is not hard work; letting our lives testify to His love and power within us was never meant to be an arduous task.

I am not saying that this is always easy and that we don't, at times, encounter opposition (and some of it most unpleasant). But the most effective witnessing is for us to share who Jesus really *is* to us rather than trying to recall what He is meant to be. I can only really give you what I have, isn't that right?

We said a lot earlier in this book that the reasons why some of us may have struggled with accusation, OCD and addictions are going to be very varied. But we share one thing in common...

Today

We all have today. Today, we can invite the Lord to, once again, take the reins of our lives. He is well able to bring us to our Kingdom purpose. None of us, of ourselves, deserve such grace, but let's receive it, nonetheless, because He offers it generously.

He is well able to break us free from shackles which would seek to keep us bound. The enemy is no longer the key holder. Jesus has the key, and at the Cross He unlocked us and transferred us from Darkness to the Kingdom of Light. We are to expect heaven on earth, Kingdom values to operate in our lives. I am not saying this will always be our experience – I hope it is or becomes yours, but at the moment it isn't mine. Yet it is more mine today than it was five years ago, even two years ago, even last year. Actually I thank Him that He has done identifiable work in my life over the last four months.

> **We cannot change yesterday...**

We cannot change yesterday, but our eternal Lord can take us from today. I believe that He does a lot more than that. He is eternal and His life-giving Spirit is now the power which has made us alive in Him. He lives outside time. So do we!

We are part of this world but do not belong to this temporary kingdom. The Holy Spirit can move in our lives *eternally*. He promises to go ahead of us, and I believe that He can straighten out and heal past issues too. Nothing is too hard for Him to handle.

Steven Furtick[15] writes:

> "Most of us give up too soon on the greater life God has for us. Don't lose hope. With God, nothing in your life is ever beyond resuscitation. And even in situations that feel wasted, wrapped in sorrow, cold to the touch, He has the power to bring forth one thousand new lives."

He wants to so fill us, so impact us with *Himself*, that other authorities in our lives cannot stand. They have to bow. Do we want them to? Do we want to break away from useless habits and burdensome addictions? He can touch our lives and make the way.

For some people miracles happen. I know of people who have come off a drug habit with no side effects at all. Others may be led to attend therapy or counselling.

I have known the direct touch of the Holy Spirit to wean me off habits that have hampered me. I have also spent time talking and praying with

---

[15] See Bibliography (p.106)

those who have been kind enough to support me. Jesus knows me and He knows you. He knows how to touch *you*. Will you let Him?

Let's ask Him.

> *Lord Jesus, I thank you that I am Yours and that You have also completely given Yourself to me. Thank you for the abundant Life that you won for me at the Cross. I acknowledge that there are areas of my life where I am not experiencing your Life; substitute loves and substitute lords have sat on the throne of areas of my life.*
>
> *As we talk now, Lord, I want to bring you the area(s) of [name it / them]. I believe that you have redeemed me from this because your victory at the Cross was complete and you included me! I was crucified with You, and I no longer live. This habit / addiction no longer lives. Your Life lives in me!*
>
> *Lord, reveal to me what You did at the Cross. Show me, Holy Spirit, how to walk out of the binding behaviours that have shackled me. I repent of them; Lord, I turn my face from them and choose to acknowledge my position in You – seated with You in heavenly places, far above all rule and authority.*
>
> *Lord, I expect to see change in my life. I expect to see my hunger for you to increase and my hunger for salty water to decrease. Holy Spirit, come and work that out through me.*
>
> *Lord Jesus, I affirm that I am trusting You. As I rest in my identity as a son, may Your abundance grow in me and may Life overcome.*
>
> *In Jesus' Name.*
>
> *Amen!*

Amen – let it be so!

Now, just feel for a moment the freedom of having given Him back the responsibility to work in ways that only He can.

19

RESOLVE

"I fear all we have done is to awaken a sleeping giant and fill him with a terrible resolve."[16]

The words attributed to the Japanese Admiral after the 1941 attack on Pearl Harbour may, or may not, have passed his lips. At the least, they depict the somewhat guarded response of a commander who sensed that his forces had failed to deliver a knockout blow to his foe; the Americans were hurt and beaten up that day, but the anxieties of their enemies who feared even greater reprisals proved to be well founded.

You and I may have taken considerable abuse at the hands of the accuser. Looking back, it may seem as if he has raided our lives, ravaged them even. Nevertheless, we may have been down but we are not out, and once again we can stand on our feet, face the Liar and begin to live from the place of authority where we have been stationed.

Do not beat yourself up, either, that you may have listened to these lies for so long. There is nothing to

Do not beat yourself up...

be gained from self-recrimination. The point, dear friend, is that your eyes are now being opened, and like the strings that held down Gulliver, you may be seeing that the ropes that have bound you are not the imprisoning fortress they appeared to be.

---

[16] Admiral Isoroku Yamamoto of the Japanese Fleet

As we have prayed in the previous chapter, God wants us to simply take His hand and walk with Him – starting *now*. I can't change the struggles I have had with OCD, but I can certainly redeem them by trusting all that has happened to Him and walking on with Him now. I have some new equipment on board too; I have learned to discern the difference between the Voice from heaven and the Pointing Finger. I have seen the fruit of them both. I know now how it feels when they speak, the effect that they have on me, the fruit that is borne in my life when I respond to them.

God knows very specifically what He has allowed to cross the threshold of your life. I remember once I was praying about part of the difficult path I have taken. He showed me a stick of rock – you know, the sticky, sweet, sugary souvenir you can buy at a British seaside. There are different flavours and thicknesses of this healthy (!) treat, but what you find throughout is the name of the seaside town piped into the rock so that it is visible from the stick's top to its end.

The stick that I saw had a thread of gold running right through the middle. You see, Jesus was showing me that nothing was going to be wasted; that everything was redeemable; that truly, all things work together for those who love God and are called according to His purposes.

I can only think that there are brothers and sisters, young and old, in the Body of Christ, who come under accusation, who are on their freedom road, and reading this book is just part of the process.

APPENDIX

HAVE YOU MET HIM YET?

As I write, the specification description on TV sets, 'HD Ready', is already superseded on many models by 'Full HD'. HD means High Definition, for the as yet uninitiated.

My own TV is HD Ready. If I were to upgrade my not-so-technical brain and find the inclination to equally upgrade my equipment, I would be able to benefit from a sharper, clearer picture.

God offers you a revolutionary upgrade to your life, whether you are satisfied with your current model or not.

May I ask you a question? Are you Heaven Destination ready?

You and I can be. We can live from a place where we are ready, in a moment, in the twinkling of an eye, to move from our present, temporary stay here on earth to a permanent Kingdom destination.

If we already have a relationship with Jesus, regardless of its potency, the fact is that we are already seated in heavenly places. Our earthly death, whenever that may occur, will merely see us transferred from one domain to another. Our physical body, having ceased to function, will mean that we can no longer live on this earth, and our spirit man will continue to live in Heaven. And it will be clothed in a new heavenly body, which will not be overweight, aching, painful, non-functioning or tired!

Nevertheless, the Lord would have us live right now from those heavenly places; this will maximise our wondrous experience of Him on earth and also, as a springtime fragrance, spread Kingdom influence here around us.

For those reading who have never invited Jesus to 'take them on' in this life and who, like the famous woman at the well (John 4), may perhaps be tired of trying to make it in this life under their own steam, please consider this opportunity to take part in an exchange. You are offered a *divine* exchange.

> **You are offered a divine exchange.**

Divine Exchange

Become Heaven ready. Cross over the bridge from a life without Christ to the Kingdom of God. Don't be tempted to 'go all holy', to pray something clever or to change your clothes or hairstyle. If you recognise that you are not living His Life and would like to, here is a chance for you.

You and I were born separated from God. Jesus bridged that separation by taking the penalty for your and my condition (and our subsequent actions) on the Cross. He paid that debt. He paid your debt whether you recognise it or not; but you need to redeem your coupon to partner in what He did.

It would be a sad waste if the coupon with your name on it remained unused or unredeemed.

So, if this resonates with you, I would like to invite you to simply and genuinely pray with me the following prayer. It may seem a small step for you, but, believe me, the step that God is taking towards you is enormous, and you are going to wonderfully discover life-changing Life.

> *Lord Jesus, I believe that You died on the Cross and shed Your Blood to settle the penalty of my separation from You. Please forgive me for all that I have done wrong, deliberately*

or otherwise. Likewise, I am ready to forgive any and all who have hurt me. As you freely forgive me, I equally release others.

I gratefully receive your forgiveness. Please come in to my life as my Lord and Saviour.

Holy Spirit, come in to my life and 'take me on'.

Jesus, You promised to make me new. Yes, come in and do that, and reveal more and more of Yourself to me through the Bible, through other Christians and through Your Holy Spirit.

Thank you, Lord Jesus. Amen.

Congratulations if you have prayed this and meant it! God has kept His side and done something supernatural in your life.

If you found it difficult to sincerely forgive someone, just bring that to Him. As you are willing, He will work in your life and help you to release those who have meant you harm. He knows everything about you (Psalm 139) and knows how to get through to you. We need to understand that forgiveness matters. Proverbs 18:19 says:

PROVERBS 18:19

"A brother offended is harder to be won than a strong city, and contentions are like the bars of a citadel."

We suffer when we do not forgive. We might think that we are holding power over the one who has offended us, but the reality is that the offence is holding us captive. Proverbs 19:8 goes on to say:

PROVERBS 19:8

"He who gets wisdom loves his own soul; he who keeps understanding will find good."

...and in verse 11:

PROVERBS 19:11

"A man's discretion makes him slow to anger, and it is his glory to overlook a transgression."

You and I are on a journey of discovering His miracle-working power in many aspects of life. But the greatest miracle is that He, upon our confession and acceptance of Him, has transferred us from one kingdom to His Kingdom.

You are Heaven Destination ready. How wonderful!

Just as hot coals need other hot coals around them to maintain their temperature, I would encourage you to seek out a friendly, Bible-believing church where the Holy Spirit is welcome to express Himself. God will help you to find a place where you can feel at home and grow in your faith. God's Spirit within you is able to work in your life and bring transformation. You will not be able to do this in your own strength, nor are you designed to attempt to do so.

As a result of your decision to align your life with the Cross and to receive Jesus, many will now rejoice with you – and a few may not.

I have a thing about scents. Smells. A barbecue, petrol, a newly surfaced road, scents in a forest or garden, fresh coffee. And I confess to taking delight in different perfumes (or shall we say *eau de toilette,* from a gent's point of view). I have quite a few. Scents are evocative, rich, invigorating, powerful. They change the immediate atmosphere around you. And that's exactly what the Holy Spirit wants to do where you are.

May I wish you every blessing in your walk with Jesus Christ, your friend, Lord and Saviour, the King of Kings and Lord of Lords!

BIBLIOGRAPHY

The Fight; John White; Inter Varsity Christian Fellowship, USA (1977)

The Devil and the Sovereignty of God; Lynda Rose; Kingsway Publications Ltd (1995)

The Nature of God; Graham Cooke; Sovereign World (2003)

Brainlock; Jeffrey M Schwartz; ReganBooks (1996)

Blood and Glory; Steve Hawkins; Creation House (2014)

The Seven Longings of the Human Heart; Mike Bickle; Forerunner Books (2006)

The Bait of Satan; John Bevere; Creation House (1994)

www.cracked.com/article_15725_the-10-steps-to-porn-addiction-where-are-you.html

www.businessinsider.com/coca-cola-vs-pepsi-timeline-2013-1?op=1

www.bankofengland.co.uk/banknotes/documents/kyb_lo_res.pdf

Greater; Steven Furtick; Multnomah Books (2012)